Providing Support at Home for Children and Young People Who Have Complex Health Needs

Providing Support at Home for Children and Young People Who Have Complex Health Needs

Jaqui Hewitt-Taylor

Bournemouth University

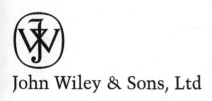

John Wiley & Sons, Ltd

Other Wiley Editorial Offices

John Wiley & Sons Inc., 111 River Street, Hoboken, NJ 07030, USA

Jossey-Bass, 989 Market Street, San Francisco, CA 94103-1741, USA

Wiley-VCH Verlag GmbH, Boschstr. 12, D-69469 Weinheim, Germany

John Wiley & Sons Australia Ltd, 42 McDougall Street, Milton, Queensland 4064, Australia

John Wiley & Sons (Asia) Pte Ltd, 2 Clementi Loop #02-01, Jin Xing Distripark, Singapore 129809

John Wily & Sons Canada Ltd, 6045 Freemont Blvd, Mississauga, ONT, L5R 4J3, Canada

Wiley also publishes its books in a variety of electronic formats. Some content that appears in print may not
be available in electronic books.

Library of Congress Cataloging-in-Publication Data:

Hewitt-Taylor, Jaqui.
   Providing support at home for children and young people who have complex health needs /
Jaqui Hewitt-Taylor.
        p. ; cm.
   Includes bibliographical references.
   ISBN 978-0-470-51731-4 (cloth : alk. paper)
   1. Chronically ill children–Home care.   2. Children with disabilities–Home care.   3. Young adults with
disabilities–Home care.   I. Title.
   [DNLM: 1. Home Care Services.   2. Adolescent.   3. Child.   4. Chronic Disease.   5. Nurse-Patient
Relations.   6. Professional-Family Relations.   WY 115 H611p 2008]
   RJ380.H494   2008
   618.92–dc22

2007043601

Library of Congress Cataloging-in-Publication Data

A catalogue record for this book is available from the British Library

ISBN 9780470517314

Typeset in 10/12.5pt Palatino by Aptara Inc., New Delhi, India

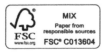

To John, my 3-year-old son.
He really did the writing, whilst I played with the
trains and diggers.

Contents

Preface   *xi*

**1 Children and Young People who have Complex and Continuing
  Health Needs**   **1**
  Definitions   1
  Providing Care at Home   4
  Economic Issues   6
  The Best Option for Individuals   7
  Achieving Home Care   8

2 Putting the Child or Young Person First   **10**
  Quality of Life   11
  The Child or Young Person's Priorities, Preferences and Choices   12
  Communication   14
  Play   18
  Social Opportunities and Leisure Activities   21
  Education   22
  The Right to Privacy   26
  Developing Independence   27
  Summary   28

3 The Child or Young Person as a Part of the Family   **29**
  Family   29
  Parenting   30
  Being the Parent of a Child who has Complex Needs   32
  Expert Parents   35
  The Impact of having a Child who has Complex Needs   37
  Social Opportunities   40
  Employment and Finances   42
  Relationships Between Parents   43
  Effects on the Family   44

The Impact of the Child's Needs on their Siblings   47
The Impact of the Child's Needs on the Extended Family   49
Summary   50

4 Working with Parents   **52**
Negotiation   52
Building Relationships   54
Respect   56
Respect for Parents' Responsibility for their Child   57
Trust   58
Boundaries in Professional Relationships   60
Working with Parents who are Experts   63
Enabling and Supporting Parents to Access and Accept Support   66
Understanding and Working with the Family's Expectations   67
Summary   69

5 Working in the Family Home   **70**
Being a Visitor in One's own Workplace   70
Intrusion Versus Support   71
Staff Safety and Well-being in the Workplace   76
Confidentiality   79
Summary   81

6 Supporting Young People   **83**
Developing Independence   83
Risk Taking   86
Developing Peer Relationships   89
Image and Identity   90
Sexuality and Sexual Expression   91
Further Education   94
Preparing for Employment   95
Transition to Adult Services   96
Summary   99

7 Grief, Loss and Bereavement   **100**
Grief and Loss for Children and Young People   100
Sources of Loss for Parents   104
Sources of Loss for other Family Members   109
Theories of Grief, Loss and Bereavement   110
Children and Young People's Concepts of Death   112

Families Living with Loss 115
Supporting Families who Experience Loss 117
Loss for Healthcare Staff 119
Summary 120

8 **Choices and Rights** **121**
Children's Rights 121
Autonomy 122
Autonomy and Healthcare 125
Competence in Decision Making 127
Consent 129
Empowerment 131
Advocacy 133
Child Protection 136
Equality and Disability Rights 138
Summary 139

9 **Ethical Issues Involved in Supporting Children, Young People and their Families** **141**
Morals and Ethics 142
Promoting Health 142
Ethical Principles 145
Duties of Healthcare Professionals 151
Fidelity 154
Responsibility 154
Summary 155

10 **Organisational Issues** **157**
Support 157
Determining what is Needed 159
Joined-up Assessment 161
Collaborative Working 162
The Key Worker 166
Organising Care Packages 167
Independent Funding Options 169
Short-Break Services 170
Summary 172

11 **Working with Children, Young People and Their Families** **174**
Seeing the Child or Young Person First 174
The Child or Young Person as a Part of their Family 176

x   *Contents*

Working in the Family Home   177
Supporting Young People   178
Decision Making and Finite Resources   179

Appendix: Useful Resources   *181*

References   *185*

Index   *199*

Preface

Children and young people who are described as having complex and continuing health needs have a variety of health related needs. Technical competence and knowledge of the child's condition are essential parts of providing them with support. However, children and their families also highly value support that shows respect for them as individuals and as families, and which demonstrates some insight into their needs as people, rather than as tasks to be completed (Hewitt-Taylor 2007).

With this in mind, this book explores some general aspects of supporting children who have complex and continuing health needs and their families in their own homes, rather than discussing specific disorders, diseases, treatments or interventions. The chapters focus on: seeing the child or young person first and foremost as a child or young person; working with and seeing the family as a whole but individual unit; working closely with parents; working in the family home; supporting young people who have complex and continuing health needs; understanding grief and loss in relation to children and young people who have complex and continuing health needs; respecting the rights of children and young people who have complex health needs; the ethical issues involved in supporting children, young people and their families; and the organisational issues involved in service provision. Case studies are used to illustrate and apply the points which are raised.

Chapter 1
Children and Young People who have Complex and Continuing Health Needs

Developments in biomedicine, technology and supportive care mean that life-threatening conditions and events which were previously considered incompatible with life (such as extremely premature birth) can now be survived. At the same time, children who have progressive diseases (for example muscular dystrophy) often have increased life expectancy (Noyes 2006a).

This ability to save and sustain life means that there are an increasing number of children and young people who require medical or technical support for many years, sometimes for their entire life, to maintain or optimise their health. Many children and young people in this situation also need substantial and ongoing care to avert death or to prevent their disabilities from worsening (Nessa 2004). Such children and young people are sometimes described as having health needs that are complex and continuing (Department of Health 2004a). As children who have complex and continuing health needs are increasingly living into adulthood, a population of young people and adults who have this type of need is now also emerging (Condliffe 2006; Shribman 2007).

DEFINITIONS

The increasing number of children and young people who have complex and continuing health needs is often referred to, but there is no absolute consensus on what constitute 'complex and continuing health needs' (Stalker et al. 2003). The phrase 'children with complex needs' is often used to refer to this group. However, this can be confusing, as the term does not relate exclusively to those with complex and continuing health needs. It includes children and young people with a variety of complex needs: those who are the subject of child protection plans; looked after children; children who are leaving care settings; children for whom adoption is planned; children with complex educational needs; young offenders; children who have significant mental health problems; and children with complex disabilities or complex health needs (Department for Education and Skills and Department of Health 2006).

The term 'complex and continuing health needs' implies that a child or young person has complex health related needs, rather than the more general term 'children with complex needs'. It also means that their health needs are expected to be sustained and are continuing over some time, rather than an acute stage of an illness. However, precisely how a child or young person is assessed as having a complex and continuing health need is not always easy to articulate.

Many of the definitions related to children and young people having complex and continuing health needs have been developed in conjunction with eligibility criteria for services. The reasons for this may include enabling service providers to ascertain what services the child or young person is likely to require or be entitled to in a relatively straightforward manner, or to account for or anticipate the need for service provision (Shenkman and Wegener 2000; Boddy et al. 2006). Such definitions may use service use alone (for example, whether or not a child or young person requires the involvement of a certain service or number of services) or a combination of service use and whether the child or young person has specific impairments (Greco and Sloper 2004; Boddy et al. 2006; Stevens 2006). One problem with this approach is that the individual concerned must already be using, or have been assessed to require, services in order to be defined as having complex and continuing health needs. A self-perpetuating cycle may be set up in this way if a child or young person is not assessed as requiring services. Because of not requiring certain services, they may not be considered to have complex and continuing health needs, which may in turn mean that they are not deemed to require certain services. It may also exclude children and young people who are awaiting assessment, or whose needs do not neatly fit a particular type of service provision.

Another approach to defining whether or not a child or young person has complex and continuing health needs is to focus on medical or physical health issues, and base the definition on their diagnosis or diagnoses (Shenkman and Wegener 2000) or the complexity of their health related needs (Boddy et al. 2006). These definitions focus very clearly on whether or not a child or young person has complex health needs, rather than other types of complex need. However, they can mean that other important needs which they have are excluded from their assessment. For example, their social and emotional needs, any behavioural difficulties that they may have and organisational aspects of support may be missed, although these may be very important to their quality of life. In addition, definitions that focus on diagnosis may exclude those children or young people who do not have, or do not yet have, a definite diagnosis and reduce their options for service provision despite having significant needs (Boddy et al. 2006).

The terms 'technology dependent' or 'dependent on technology' have also been used to describe some children and young people who have complex and continuing health needs (Noyes 2006b). These terms provide considerable clarity over the child or young person's needs and over what aspects and types of medical or technical assistance they require (for example, assisted ventilation, continuous positive airways pressure). Nonetheless, like the definitions that focus on the child or young person's physical or medical needs, they may mean that support becomes focused on medical or technical needs, rather than seeing the child or young person and their family holistically.

Another option is to base assessment on the child or young person's individual needs, and decide on a case-by-case basis whether they have health needs that are complex and continuing. This allows service providers the opportunity to place the person, not just their diagnosis, physical or medical needs, or service use, centrally (Boddy et al. 2006). However, whilst it fulfils the ideal of seeing the child or young person holistically and humanistically, it may be problematic in any situation in which numbers and predefined or standardised criteria are required to account for the use of resources.

The debate over the definition of a child or young person who has complex and continuing health needs illustrates the difficulty that can be experienced in seeing the child or young person and their family holistically, when service provision and decisions as to which service will fund aspects of support needs to be accounted for. One of the problems with attempting to define what constitutes a child or young person who has complex and continuing health needs is that this tends to categorise people in a way which can be unhelpful (Boddy et al. 2006). Whilst ostensibly creating a mechanism to provide children, young people and their families with support, it may predispose to that support being organised and delivered in a way that devalues people as individuals and focuses on tasks or discrete needs. A vital aspect of working with children and young people who have complex and continuing health needs and their families is to acknowledge, but see beyond, these needs to the person and people involved (Leonardi et al. 2006).

The complexity of defining whether or not a child or young person is defined as having complex and continuing health needs means that precisely how many children and young people have this type of need is difficult to determine (Glendinning and Kirk 2000). However, there are now estimated to be as many as 6000 children in the United Kingdom living at home, but dependent on technology to meet their health needs and sustain their lives (Shribman 2007).

PROVIDING CARE AT HOME

There has, for many years, been a trend in The United Kingdom for health related care and support to be delivered in the home, rather than hospital or institutional settings, wherever possible (Department of Health 1990). There has also been a sustained move towards enabling all people who have long-term conditions to live at home, and to develop and improve the services that people receive when their health and social care needs are met in the community (Department of Health 2006).

As well as a general move towards providing community, rather than hospital based care, avoiding children being hospitalised unnecessarily has been on the British policy agenda since the late 1950s, with the Platt Report (Platt 1959) often cited as an early instrument of implementing this aim. Ongoing recommendations, such the Court Report (Commission of Child Health Services 1976) and the Audit Commission (1993) report have continued to identify that children should only be cared for in hospital when this has a therapeutic advantage over home care. This approach has more recently been advocated in the National Service Framework for children, young people and maternity services (Department of Health 2004a).

The move away from children being hospitalised has been largely attributed to consideration of the child and family's well-being. It has been suggested that children's emotional, psychological, developmental, educational, and social needs are generally better met at home than in hospital (Balling and McCubbin 2001; Neufeld et al. 2001). There is also some evidence that the physical health of children who have complex health needs is improved when they are cared for at home compared with when they are cared for in hospital (Appierto et al. 2002).

The philosophy of enabling children to remain at home, rather than in hospital or institutional settings wherever possible applies equally to children and young people who have complex and continuing health needs. This nonetheless represents a significant change from the way in which their care was traditionally provided. Children and young people who have this type of need would once have spent prolonged periods of time in hospital, in some cases their entire lives (Kirk et al. 2005). Where they required assisted ventilation this would have included long periods of time being spent in an intensive care unit. However, it has been recognised for some time that intensive care units are not appropriate places for children and young people who require long-term assisted ventilation but are otherwise medically stable to be cared for (Department of Health 1998).

The intensive care environment is not conducive to a child or young person's development, because intensive care units are primarily designed for sustaining life in acute situations. Children and young people who spend prolonged periods of time on an intensive care unit will usually be exposed to sights, sounds and disturbances to their day that are not developmentally or emotionally beneficial. Their daytime routines and sleep are likely to be disturbed, and the children around them will not normally be able to play and interact with them. Although parents are welcomed on paediatric intensive care units, they are usually unable to maintain the natural contact with their child that they would have in the family home and their privacy is very limited. The child's mobility is usually constrained by the environment if not by their physical needs, as they are not free to explore intensive care units as they would be their home environment. Their ability to access education, visit and be visited by family and friends is also likely to be limited by their location.

Where the competing demands on paediatric intensive care staff include carrying out life-saving and preserving interventions, providing a full range of developmental experiences for a child or young person who is medically stable is unlikely to always hold the highest priority. It is therefore almost inevitable that children who are cared for long term in an intensive care unit will be exposed to inappropriate levels of stimulation and will not enjoy the same developmental experiences enjoyed by other children or young people of their age (Boosfeld and O'Toole 2000).

An acute hospital setting is also an inappropriate place for children to grow up in. Although the other children and young people in hospital wards are not usually as acutely or critically ill as those on intensive care units, they are unlikely to provide the type of peer relationships that children and young people would usually experience. Children are also unlikely to have the same range of experiences or interactions with adults that they would encounter at home. The number of staff who care for children in hospital and their varied views on child rearing makes establishing consistent practices problematic. Although parents often provide for the majority of their child's day-to-day care on hospital wards, they effectively 'parent in public' and have very limited privacy, both for establishing and maintaining a relationship with their child and for conducting their own relationships.

Caring for their child whilst they are in hospital can place a much greater burden on parents than caring for their child at home. Travelling to and from hospital means that juggling the visiting and care of the child in hospital, with the rest of their lives is very difficult. If the family have other children, parents' contact with them and the child's contact with their siblings will be disrupted when one child is hospitalised long term. Similarly, relationships between parents and with other family members and friends may be affected and parents may have relatively little opportunity for social support. Friends and relatives may have to travel a greater distance than they otherwise would to visit the child, and restrictions on visiting can mean that the child and their parents cannot see groups of their family or friends together.

Taylor (2000) also suggests that children, young people and their families are generally provided with better information when their care is provided outside the hospital environment. It is also possible that parents will be in a more powerful position at home than they would be in hospital. In hospital, healthcare staff are often seen as holding more power than parents, and parents are visitors in an unfamiliar environment. This situation is somewhat reversed in the family home, as healthcare staff are the visitors and have a greater obligation to respect the family's rules, values, norms and ownership of their child (Farasat and Hewitt-Taylor 2007). As Chapter 5 discusses, this does not mean that parents will necessarily find having a child who has complex health needs living at home an empowering experience. However, it may be less disempowering than their child being in hospital long term.

Despite the general acceptance of the ideal of organising healthcare to enable children and young people to remain at home, it is also important to note that there is a relatively weak research base to support the move to home care. It is more likely that this has been popularised and developed because of its intuitive appeal to the public and professionals (Parker et al. 2006).

ECONOMIC ISSUES

Although the benefits that children, young people and their families can derive from home care are often cited, there are also a financial and organisational incentives for support to be provided to enable children and young people who have complex and continuing health needs to live at home. Appierto et al. (2002) suggest that care at home is the most cost effective option for children with complex and continuing health needs. Providing hospital based care for them has been described as an inappropriate use of resources, both in financial terms and in terms of use of acute care facilities (Boosfeld and O'Toole 2000). The increasing population of such children and young people is one which the availability of acute beds, particularly paediatric intensive care beds, and staffing cannot support. However, although it is generally suggested that home care is a cheaper option for service providers, Noyes et al. (2006) identify that this is mostly, but not always, the case when the child or young person requires long-term assisted ventilation. There are circumstances where hospital based care for some children or young people who require long-term technical intervention is less costly, particularly if they are housed outside an intensive care setting.

Another consideration with cost estimates is that whilst home care may be the most cost-effective option for the National Health Service, it may move some of the financial burden of caring for children with complex and continuing health needs from the National Health Service to the families concerned (O'Brien and Wegner 2002). Having a child who has complex and continuing health needs is often very costly, financially, for their families (O'Brien and Wegner 2002; Parker et al. 2006). Whilst the cost of home care (for example, funding for equipment, staffing and supplies) may be met by the NHS and Social Services, the family usually incur many incidental expenses. It is estimated that the cost of bringing up a disabled child is three times higher than bringing up a child who is not disabled (Department of Health 2004a). This cost is likely to be even greater where the child has complex and continuing health needs. The costs that parents incur may include: providing transport for their child; buying toys that their child can use (which are often more expensive than other toys); obtaining specialist furniture; providing electricity to power the devices which they use; and the numerous telephone calls which they have to make (Hewitt-Taylor 2007). Many parents' ability to remain in employment and the type of employment in which they can engage is adversely affected by having a child who has complex and continuing health needs (Hewitt-Taylor 2007). This often means that families have a lower income whilst their outgoing expenses are increased (Department of Health 2004a).

The expenses associated with a child being hospitalised long term have not been formally compared with the expenses incurred by families when a child is cared for at home. It is nonetheless clear that having a child who has complex and continuing health needs is expensive in comparison to a child who does not have this type of need. In addition, not all the costs incurred by parents as a result of their child's health needs are met by service providers or state benefits.

THE BEST OPTION FOR INDIVIDUALS

The assumption is generally that enabling children and young people to live at home is the most desirable option. However, this will not always be the case. As well as the financial cost that parents incur when they have a child who has complex health needs living at home, there is considerable responsibility and work placed on the whole family (Parker et al. 2006; Hewitt-Taylor 2007). Where a child has the type of needs that require daily, continuing and demanding care provision, the cost in physical, social and emotional terms for a family may be a burden which they are unable to bear, despite ideally wanting their child to be at home (Carnevale et al. 2006; Parker et al. 2006).

When decisions are made regarding where and by whom a child with complex and continuing health needs is cared for and will live, the needs of the whole family should be taken into account, and who will benefit and whose benefit is the most important considered (Hewitt-Taylor 2007). These are potentially difficult and emotionally charged decisions, and include not only the child's quality of life but their parents' quality of life, the quality of life of any siblings, and how these will impact on one another. Although the child's well-being is paramount in all decisions concerning them (Department of Health 2004b), every child's well-being, including that of siblings, and how parents' well-being will impact on their children's well-being must be included in the decision making process.

Although home care is, in principle, the best option, what is best will not be the same for every child or family. For some children and families, caring for their child at home is not the best option. Where this decision is reached, the family should be offered support to help them to live with the difficult decisions that they have made, and to continue to have meaningful and rewarding input into their child's life (Parker et al. 2006). Where home care is the best option, support to enable children, young people and their families to achieve the best possible quality of life needs to be put in place.

ACHIEVING HOME CARE

When it is decided that a child or young person who has complex and continuing health needs will live at home, setting up the services which will enable them to be discharged from hospital can be a protracted process (Department of Health 2004a). In addition, whilst the initial setting up of the services required may be difficult to effect, equally important and potentially problematic is ensuring that the ongoing support which children and their families need is in place (Department of Health 2004a; Brazier 2006).

In order to facilitate the child or young persons' discharge from hospital, and to provide effective support for them and their families once they are at home, careful planning, co-ordination and co-operation between services is needed. This necessitates a comprehensive assessment of the child or young person's needs, including their medical, technical, social, emotional and educational needs and the needs of their family. Funding, responsibilities for various aspects of support, and governance frameworks must all be agreed. A range of health, social care and education providers and professionals at managerial and individual level are likely to be involved in establishing home care, and all need to work in a co-ordinated and co-operative manner if this is to be achieved smoothly and to a high standard.

Facilitating home care provision requires staff who are able to support children and their families during the discharge process, but also following their discharge home. When it becomes clear that a child will require long-term health related intervention and home care is the goal, a team of staff must often be provided who can assist the child and family on a day-to-day basis. This frequently includes needs or services that span both health and social care provision. From the healthcare perspective, an NHS or Primary Care Trust is often not in a position to have a bank of staff employed awaiting such a need to arise. This means that families must often wait whilst decisions are made as to how and by whom support will be provided, and in many cases whilst staff are recruited and trained to assist them. Recruiting and retaining staff to fulfil such roles is often difficult and significant delays in a child or young person who has complex health needs being discharged home often occur because of the need for staff to be recruited to support them (Hewitt-Taylor 2007).

In addition to staff having to be recruited and trained, parents often have to develop new skills and knowledge related to their child's requirements and need the opportunity to develop confidence in these before they take their child home (Boosfeld and O'Toole 2000; Department of Health 2004a). As well as developing practical skills and knowledge, parents need to be given the chance to consider, and be supported, in accommodating the emotional workload of caring for a child who has complex and continuing health needs. This includes having to perform tasks which contrast with their expected parenting role, and which are unpleasant and distressing for them and their children (Abbott et al. 2005; Kirk et al. 2005). This can again take some time and requires staff to be available to work with and support parents who are preparing to take their child home.

The aim of enabling children who have complex and continuing health needs to live at home should be to facilitate them and their families achieving as good a quality of life as possible. For this to happen, the staff who support them need to have some insight into their needs as people, not just knowledge and skills in the medical or technical aspects of their care.

Chapter 2
Putting the Child or Young Person First

Children and young people who have complex and continuing health needs are, first and foremost, children and young people, with the same needs and rights that their peers have, and should be seen as such (Department of Health 2004a; Whitehurst 2006). However, Landsman (2005) suggests that society often sees them primarily in relation to their health needs, which tends to medicalise them, and devalue them as people.

Effective and high-quality support must obviously meet the medical or technical needs that a child or young person has. However, it needs to go beyond this. Support should be directed at enabling children and young people to enjoy the same rights and opportunities as their peers, and to reach their full potential in every area of their life (Department of Health 2004a). The United Nations Convention on the Rights of the Child (Article 23) states that disabled children should be enabled to:

> enjoy full and decent lives, in conditions which ensure dignity, promote self-reliance and facilitate the child's active participation in the community. (Office of the United Nations High Commissioner for Human Rights 1989)

The support that is provided for children and young people who have complex and continuing health needs should aim to facilitate the achievement of these rights. On a day-to-day basis, this means seeking to enable children and young people to do the things that are important to them, and to provide support which assists them to achieve what matters to them. Every person has different priorities, preferences, aspirations and values. The support that children and young people are provided with should focus on meeting their needs as perceived by them, not by others.

QUALITY OF LIFE

Enabling children and young people to achieve as good as possible a quality of life, as defined by them, should be a central aim of the support with which they are provided. Quality of life is affected by many factors, including: a persons' physical well-being, their emotional well-being, their material well-being, the interpersonal aspects of their life, their degree of self-determination, the extent to which they can achieve social inclusion, and the rights they are afforded (Schalock et al. 2002). Individuals' perceptions of quality of life are also influenced by their spiritual, cultural and personal perspectives on health and illness (Kelly and Uddin 2005).

Quality of life is therefore multifaceted, and involves a great deal more than physical health. What will create good quality of life is a very individual concept, because what each individual sees as important in achieving this varies considerably, and may change over time. For example, for some individuals material well-being is very important, whereas for others this holds a lower ranking. For some physical well-being will be more important than for others. A child or young person who has complex and continuing health needs is likely to define good physical health differently to those who do not have such needs. What will enable each individual to achieve quality of life will therefore differ, and support which is meaningful and helpful to each person can only be determined by ascertaining what matters to them.

Case study

Joanna is 15. She sustained a high spinal injury when she was seven. She has a tracheostomy, requires assisted ventilation, and communicates by others lip-reading her or by using an electronic communication device. She is dependent on other people for all her physical care.

Joanna lives with her mother, Caroline, and her sister, Anna, who is 17. She has a carer with her every night, from 10 pm until 7 am. On weekdays, she also has a carer to help her to get up, accompany her to school, be with her at school, and escort her home. Her family provide for her needs at all other times, except for 10 hours a week, for which she receives Direct Payment funding from Social Services, used to employ carers to enable her to enjoy some social activities.

Joanna enjoys goes shopping, especially for clothes and make-up. She likes spending time with other people of her age, joining her group of friends to 'just be together, chatting, listening to music, watching TV and stuff like that'. She also likes chatting online to her peers.

Although she has considerable health needs, Joanna prefers to be with and make friends amongst her nondisabled peers. She sees herself as generally in good health, has rarely been hospitalised since her initial accident, and comments that 'I hardly ever have a day off school because of being ill'.

Joanna enjoys watching television programmes about travel, and would like to have the opportunity to go travelling when she leaves school, as many of her friends are planning to do. She wonders whether there is any way this can be achieved. At present, because of funding and staffing issues, she has not been able to go on holiday since her accident, even within the UK. The family occasionally go to stay with Joanna's aunt, who lives 60 miles from their home.

When she leaves school, Joanna would like to go to university, with the aim of working in either the fashion or travel industry after graduating.

THE CHILD OR YOUNG PERSON'S PRIORITIES, PREFERENCES AND CHOICES

If a child or young person is to fulfil their potential and achieve what they consider to be the best possible quality of life, what matters most to them must be determined. For this to be achieved, it seems obvious that they need to be involved in the decisions that are made about them and the support which they receive (Cavet and Sloper 2004). Children and young people who have complex and continuing health needs, like other people, have knowledge about themselves, their feelings, values and priorities. Knowing these is essential to any decision making about service provision if this is to meet their needs (Department of Health 2004a). However, although involving children and young people in decision making about their lives is agreed in principle to be essential, and there are examples of good practice in this respect, there is also evidence that it does not always occur (Cavet and Sloper 2004).

Children and young people should be involved in the decisions that are made about all aspects of their lives, and enabled to make real choices about the same spectrum of activities that any other child or young person can. This includes small, but extremely significant, day-to-day events being planned and carried out in accordance with their preferences. In most cases, and perhaps especially when a child or young person cannot communicate verbally, staff working with them consistently is an important part of this. It affords both parties the opportunity to develop a relationship with one another, to learn how to communicate effectively with one another, for staff to begin to understand what the child or young person's condition means to them, and what their values, preferences and priorities are. Staff knowing the child or young person in this way can be a significant step to enabling them to live, day to day, as they would prefer.

Case study

Joanna has very definite views on how her hair and make-up should be done, and on what she wears. Going to school 'looking good' is very important to her. However, the carers who support Joanna vary in their ability to 'do' make-up and hair styling. Joanna has asked whether it is possible for certain carers who are good at, and enjoy, this aspect of her care, to be available to get her up and ready for school during the week (at weekends her mother helps her get up and her older sister does her hair and make-up). Although the team who support her try to facilitate this, it is not always possible. Joanna dreads the days when she knows she will go to school looking 'a mess'. She explains: 'I never have time off school, but once or twice I have wondered about skiving off, because I was like "I can't go to school, looking like this."'

Because Joanna finds speaking difficult, she relies on her carers taking the time to find out exactly how she wants her hair and make-up done. She explains that, from her point of view, if they do not it means: 'They don't care about me. I don't believe they really can't learn it. They all learn how to do my ventilator, and trache, so how come they can't learn to do my hair? They could learn, they just don't see it as important. They aren't the ones stuck at school looking a mess.'

The extent to which what is termed 'involvement' in decisions about their lives truly involves children and young people is variable. It can mean: being supported to express their views; being listened to; their views being taken into account in decision making; being involved in decision-making processes and influencing the outcome of these; and sharing power in and responsibility for decision making (Shier 2001). It is important that involving children and young people in decision making includes action being taken on their views, rather than these only being listened to. This may be complicated and time consuming, but as Whitehurst (2006) identifies, unless it occurs, children and young people will only be 'done unto' and the support with which they are provided may not enhance, and may even detract from, the quality of their life.

Individual staff may be very effective at listening to children and young people's preferences and basing their day-to-day care and support on these. However, unless service provision is also based on their views and priorities, there will still be limits to their achieving quality of life. Therefore, mechanisms by which the views of children and young people provide influence beyond their day-to-day care provision need to be put in place. This extends to their opinions being included in local and national policy.

Although the quality of the day-to-day support that children and young people receive is vital, it is also important for the ethos of service provision to be one which places the child or young person as an individual centrally. A major part of achieving this is enabling children and young people to express their views.

COMMUNICATION

All children have the right to be enabled and permitted to communicate. The United Nations Convention on the Rights of the Child (Article 13) states that:

> The child shall have the right to freedom of expression; this right shall include freedom to seek, receive and impart information and ideas of all kinds ... either orally, in writing or in print, in the form of art, or through any other media of the child's choice. (Office of the United Nations High Commissioner for Human Rights 1989).

Children and young people who have complex health needs, like their peers, have this right, and those seeking to support them are responsible for facilitating ways in which this right can be upheld.

Communication is essentially a process of sending and receiving messages. Broadly speaking, it is composed of two dimensions: verbal and nonverbal communication. Verbal communication is defined as spoken communication, whilst nonverbal communication is usually understood as the process of sending and receiving wordless messages. Whether written language is included in verbal or nonverbal communication is debatable, as it involves the use of words, but not spoken words. However, for practical purposes what is important is to consider the range of ways in which an individual can communicate.

The spoken word includes not only the words that are spoken, but the tone, pitch, emphasis and volume of speech. Nonverbal means of communication include the use of sight, smell, gestures, movement, posture, positions, touch, facial expressions and eye contact. The use of personal space can also constitute a form of nonverbal communication and a person's appearance can be a way of them communicating nonverbally. Individual culture, beliefs and values can affect the way people communicate and the meaning of given verbal or nonverbal statements. For example, in some cultures touch is used more extensively and with less reserve than in others and the way in which personal space is used and interpreted can differ between cultures.

The process of learning to communicate begins in infancy. Babies start to communicate from their first cry and very quickly produce a range of sounds, postures and facial expressions that convey messages. They learn to use their senses to detect changes in the environment, to know when other people are present, and to learn about other people's communication with them, through touch, sounds, holding and facial expressions. This process of developing one's communication skills continues and is refined throughout a person's life.

The exact mechanisms by which communication skills are acquired and refined is debated, but, despite its complexity, is something that many children acquire with no explicit teaching. However, for children and young people who have complex and continuing health needs, learning to communicate can present a challenge. This may be both because of difficulties in inputting communications from those around them and in outputting their own communications. Where a child or young person has an accident or illness that alters their communication abilities, they often have to relearn the skills which they had acquired, in a new way.

Children and young people who have complex and continuing heath needs may not receive cues and messages from others as their peers do. They may be unable to hear other people speak or move, and may have to depend on touch to know that someone is nearby or wants to gain their attention. They may be unable to see other people's facial movements and gestures, or may be unable to turn to see if a conversation or event is happening to the periphery of their visual field. They may be unable to feel sensations as well as others can, and thus may not perceive and respond to touch in the same way that others do. At the same time, many parents whose children have altered communication pathways report that their children develop alternative methods of identifying messages from others and become highly intuitive, for example, to other people being present in a room or to the emotions of those around them (Hewitt-Taylor 2007).

Some children and young people cannot use their voice to communicate their needs and preferences and have to learn alternative methods of 'speaking'. They may also be unable to use nonverbal communication such as gesture, movement, touch and posture in the way that their peers can to give emphasis or meaning to their words. In addition, they may rely on others to assist them to achieve the physical distance they prefer from those with whom they are communicating.

Children and young people who have complex health needs may have the chance to communicate with fewer people than their peers, as there may be a limit to those who understand or are prepared to make the effort to understand their way of communicating. Their restricted mobility may also lessen their opportunities to interact with a range of individuals and the spontaneity of those interactions. Other people failing to respond to a child or young person's attempts to communicate with them can also discourage them from continuing to make the effort required to interact with others. This can further impair the development of their communication skills, and their confidence in communicating and forming relationships with others.

Barriers to children and young people being enabled to communicate may include practicalities, such as whether the funding and organisation of services prioritises communication. For example, they may not have access to communication systems at both home and school, and this limits their ability to interact in at least one location. The systems which they use to communicate may be bulky or unwieldy and may be difficult for them to carry with them to use in every setting. It may also be that the funding for and allocation of human resources (such as investment in or availability of skilled workers and continuity of care provision) does not take into account the need for children and young people to be enabled to communicate. In many cases children and young people communicate using very subtle signs, and the way in which support is provided should enable relationships to be developed that facilitate this type of communication (Regnard et al. 2007). In addition, if children and young people are to be enabled to communicate about their feelings, aspirations and preferences, trusting relationships need to develop and adequate time be available so that they feel comfortable to engage in this type of discussion (Abbott et al. 2005).

A variety of systems may be used to assist children and young people who have complex health needs to communicate. Whatever the method used to enable a child or young person to communicate is, the mainstay of facilitating communication is that individuals should be given optimum opportunities to communicate, and that their communication experiences should be rewarding (Bradshaw 1998). A major influence on whether or not children and young people who have complex health needs are able to communicate is the priority which others place on facilitating this.

Case study

Joanna has very limited speech as she finds it hard to co-ordinate this and her assisted ventilation. She relies on other people lip-reading her or on them being able and willing to use her communication aid with her. She is very sociable and wants to be involved in conversations, but she finds that people often speak to her carer instead of her. Sometimes they speak at length to her carer, without acknowledging her presence, and then: 'suddenly say "hello", and wave at me, as if I had just got here'. Joanna finds that many people either come much closer to her than they would another person or speak loudly and clearly, as if it was she, not they, who had to lip-read.

Sometimes, conversations about Joanna are held above her physical level, 'As if I wasn't here.' Recently she and her mother met an acquaintance in the street. The acquaintance chatted to Caroline without acknowledging Joanna's presence, and then asked how Caroline was planning for when Joanna finished school. Caroline directed the question to Joanna, who used her communication aid to say that she wanted to go to university and study design. Joanna recalls: 'That seemed to surprise her. That I might want to say what I want to do. Mum is great like that, she always tells people to ask me.'

When Joanna wants to join in a discussion, she cannot naturally break into a conversation as her peers can. She relies on others being sensitive to her, noticing that she wants to speak (often by her eye movements or facial expressions, and sometimes by her carer alerting her peers to this). This can mean that by the time she is able to speak, the best moment to interject is lost. Sometimes she cannot join in at all, if a discussion is moving very fast. Despite being a part of the group, she still feels peripheral because she cannot contribute as her peers can. She explains: 'Sometimes I feel as if I look a bit slow. I can think as fast as them but I can't just butt in and say my piece. That's why I quite like online chat, because I can talk almost as fast as some of the others can.'

Whilst many children and young people who have complex and continuing health needs have altered communication pathways, these are often unrelated to their cognitive functioning. It is therefore vital to distinguish the ability to speak from the ability to understand, have opinions, and want to make choices. Some children and young people who have complex and continuing health needs may nonetheless be unused to expressing their views and making choices because they have never been given the opportunity to do so. As well as providing opportunities for children and young people who have complex health needs to express themselves, those who work with them may therefore need to enable them to gain confidence in expressing their choices and preferences (Cavet and Sloper 2004). To this end, it may be valuable to facilitate their access to advocacy services to enable and support them to make choices, and to increase their confidence and abilities in expressing their views and preferences (Department of Health 2001a; Cavet and Sloper 2004). (Advocacy is discussed further in Chapter 6 in relation to supporting young people and in Chapter 8 in relation to children and young people's rights.)

Although practicalities and the way in which services are organised may impact on the opportunities that children and young people who have complex health needs have to communicate, perhaps the most important facilitators or detractors from communication are the attitudes and values of individuals and society. People feeling that they do not have time to communicate with children and young people who have complex health needs, and a belief that this is not a priority may be the greatest barrier to facilitating effective communication. This may therefore also be one of the greatest barriers to ascertaining and acting on children and young peoples' wishes and views and thus to providing them with high-quality support.

PLAY

Play is a child's natural activity and a vital part of every child's life (Skar 2002). The United Nations Convention on the Rights of the Child (Article 31) identifies that all children have the right to rest and leisure, and to engage in play and recreational activities appropriate to their age (Office of the United Nations High Commissioner for Human Rights 1989). This is equally the right of children and young people who have complex and continuing health needs, although others may have to assist and enable them to achieve their rights in this respect.

Play is an important means by which children learn about themselves, their world, and other people. It enables them to develop a range of skills and a child's ability to engage in play can therefore affect a variety of their developmental experiences, opportunities and achievements. This includes their emotional development, motor development, social development, and the development of communication skills (Mulligan 2003; Sturgess 2003; Sussenberger 2003; Pierce and Marshall 2004).

Although children who have complex health needs have the same right to and need for play as any other child, there are many barriers to them achieving this right. Problems with mobility may impede them from spontaneously engaging in play. Being unable to spontaneously select and pick up objects to examine and experiment with them may alter an infant or child's development of sensory perceptions and awareness of the effect of movement on objects (Skar 2002). A child who has a motor disability is likely to need assistance to explore their environment, which may affect the development of spatial perception. A child who is unable to reach and out and select the toys they want is not only less able to explore their environment, they are also unable to use the play activity selected to develop their motor skills. In addition, a child who cannot move freely cannot spontaneously and independently select which activity they want to engage in or which child they wish to play with as another child might. Children's ability to play may also depend on any aids to mobility or technical aids which assist them in play activities being available in all the places where they will be. Where children are dependent on others to respond to cues which indicate that they wish to engage in an activity, the extent to which others are willing and able to communicate with them influences their opportunities to play.

Children who have complex health needs may need to have an adult with them when they play. This can mean that they do not have the chance to develop independence through play and to develop independent relationships with other children in the way that their peers do (Skar 2002). They may also be unable to engage in the learning of norms associated with sharing toys that other children do, as they need another person to obtain or be involved in the negotiation of the acquisition of toys on their behalf.

Children who have complex health needs may be unable to access the same range of play and developmental activities as their peers because of limited availability. Some toys which they would enjoy using may be physically unsuitable, because they are too heavy, too bulky or because they are too difficult to manipulate. Equivalent items or activities may not be available in a model that they can use. Even basic toys often require greater consideration when the user will be a child who has complex health needs than would be required for another child. Toys that they can use are often more specialised and expensive, and less widely available than other toys (Hewitt-Taylor 2007).

As well as the effect that any physical disability has on a child's play activities, the way in which environments are designed can affect their opportunities to play. For example, playgrounds that are inaccessible for children who use wheelchairs reduce their ability to engage in play activities and to develop peer relationships (Skar 2002). Even when a play area is itself accessible, many pieces of playground equipment are not designed with children with mobility problems in mind (Hewitt-Taylor 2007). As well as reducing the child's play and development opportunities, Skar (2002) suggests that play environments which do not meet disabled children's needs can make them feel unwelcome, exclude them and make them feel devalued.

Case study

Andrew is six. He has cerebral palsy, is unable to walk and has limited movement in his arms. He can speak, but his speech is not very clear, and other people often have difficulty in understanding him.

Andrew enjoys playing in the company of other children. However, his parents, Paula and Henry, or his carer, have to help him to get the toys with which he wants to play. They also usually negotiate with other children about Andrew joining their play and using shared toys, rather than Andrew doing this, as his peers find Andrew's speech difficult to understand. When his peers change their activities, Andrew, assisted by one of his parents or a carer, uses a wheelchair to join them in any new location, which often means that he joins the game later than the other children. He can be positioned so that he is with the group, but cannot move around a game or activity as his peers can.

Andrew loves mechanical things, and spends a lot of time trying to understand how things work. However, he is unable to use many toys that require manual dexterity and cannot lift anything very heavy. His parents have bought him some computer games and activities that let him do this kind of thing, which he enjoys very much (these cost considerably more than construction toys would), but he cannot get the feel of the three-dimensional effects of the objects which he manipulates on-screen. Sometimes people try to give him light bricks to build with, but he finds these boring. He wants to see how more complex machinery works.

At weekends, Andrew likes to spend time with his older brother, David, aged 8, and his younger sister, Sara who is 4. However, the playgrounds near his home do not have good access for wheelchairs, and the slides, swings and roundabouts are not suitable for him. At a park 10 miles away there are accessible swings that are suitable for him to be in with his siblings and roundabouts which he can go on in his wheelchair. Having to travel so far is not logistically possible, and usually he watches his siblings at the playground instead of playing himself. If the weather is cold he does not go, because it would be too cold for him to sit and watch for long and this would curtail his sibling's enjoyment of their play.

At home, Andrew enjoys playing with David and Sara. However, the toys he can use are fairly limited. He is very imaginative, but he needs toys that are lightweight and which he can easily manoeuvre. He also has to have toys at the right height for him and which he can sit comfortably to use, so play activities have to be set up and prepared with his needs in mind. This means that he misses out on a lot of his siblings' spontaneous play. He enjoys being outside with his siblings, but this means Paula or Henry putting matting on the ground so he can lie or sit safely and comfortably, and making sure that he is positioned appropriately. This can take at least 30 minutes to set up. Last weekend, he wanted to watch his sister and brother play football outside and be the referee. By the time things were ready, it was raining and he had to stay indoors.

Whilst children who have complex health needs may be able to make choices regarding their play, they often have to rely on others to enable them to fulfil these. As with communication, there are many practical issues that need to be considered in facilitating play opportunities for children who have complex health needs. Similarly, a major obstacle to children being able to engage in play and leisure activities is a failure of individuals and society to recognise the right that every child has to play, and service providers and individuals not prioritising children's opportunities for play. There may also be confusion between a child's physical development or ability and their cognitive development. Play activities need to be appropriate to the child's cognitive level, as well as to their physical abilities and to be stimulating and enjoyable.

SOCIAL OPPORTUNITIES AND LEISURE ACTIVITIES

Children and young people who have complex health needs do not want to be left out of their peers' activities any more than other children or young people do. They want to have friends of the same age as them, who share similar interests, and to be able to do the things that other children and young people of their age do (Department of Health 2004a; Watson et al. 2006). They want to be safe from harassment and bullying, and to live in a society where they do not face prejudice (Department of Health 2004a).

Children and young people who have additional healthcare needs like and dislike similar things to other children of their age, such as listening to music, watching TV, shopping and playing. The difference is that whereas other children take such activities for granted, they may need considerable support, assistance and consideration by others to enable them to participate (Watson et al. 2006). The Department of Health (2004a) identifies that if they are not able to join in activities with their peers, disabled children and young people often become isolated, lonely and miss out on activities that are fun, and provide opportunities for them to make friends and learn new skills.

Enabling children and young people who have complex health needs to be included with their peers in social and leisure activities also enables other children and young people to become familiar with their needs. This may be an important step in achieving a more informed, inclusive and tolerant society. It is therefore important for children and young people who have complex health needs to be enabled to enjoy the opportunities for leisure and social activities which their peers have and to be included with them in these. However, there are many barriers to this being achieved (Department of Health 2004a).

As identified in Chapter 1, having a disabled child tends to reduce a family's income and the cost of meeting their child's needs is generally higher for their parents than for other parents (Department of Health 2004a). This may impact on what families can afford for their children to do. At the same time, the cost of children and young people who have complex health needs engaging in leisure activities may also be higher. A lack of leisure activities which this group of children and young people can access means that they often have to use specialist services away from their immediate neighbourhood. Their engagement in leisure activities can be further hampered by a lack of accessible transport to areas where such facilities do exist (Department of Health 2004a). Thus, even where facilities exist, children and young people may be unable to reach them or it may be very costly for them to do so, as families may have to pay for their transport, and for them to be accompanied by a parent or carer.

As well as increasing the cost of leisure activities, lack of accessible facilities in their neighbourhood can mean that children and young people who have complex health needs do not have the chance to socialise with their local peer group in the way that other children and young people do (Department of Health 2004a). This may mean that they have less choice of friends, and that their friends all live outside the local area. In addition, having to use specialist services often means that children and young people who have complex health needs do not have opportunities to play and socialise with nondisabled children and young people (Department of Health 2004a).

Case study

Joanna enjoys being with her peers, and they are generally very keen to include her in their activities. She attends a local school, and likes to join her friends who live nearby when they walk to school. Her carer finishes work at 4 pm on weekdays, and this means that although Joanna can travel home with her peers, if they decide to go shopping, or go to the local park after school, she cannot join them.

In the evenings and at weekends, unless she has a carer booked as part of her 10 hours Direct Payments or unless her sister or her mother can go with her, Joanna cannot meet her friends. Although the 10 hours of Direct Payments she receives do enable her to go out, Joanna cannot make spontaneous decisions about social events as her peers can as these have to be planned and staff booked in advance. When she goes out with her sister or mother as her carer, she feels that she is more constrained than her peers, because one of her family is present, and her peers are also more guarded in their discussions, because: 'someone else's Mum is there'.

EDUCATION

All children have a right to education (Office of the United Nations High Commissioner for Human Rights 1989). It plays a pivotal role in their lives and should encompass more than just the quest for academic achievement (Russell 2003). The United Nations Convention on the Rights of the Child (Article 29) states that education should be directed towards:

The development of the child's personality, talents, mental and physical abilities to their fullest potential

and:

The preparation of the child for responsible life in a free society, in the spirit of understanding, peace, tolerance, equality of sexes, and friendship among all peoples, ethnic, national and religious groups and persons of indigenous origin. (Office of the United Nations High Commissioner for Human Rights 1989)

Children and young people who have complex and continuing health needs have the same right to education as other children, and the breadth of experience that education should offer applies equally to them (Berry and Dawkins 2004). If a child or young person cannot attend school or college, this may not only affect their ability to learn and develop new skills and knowledge, but reduces their chances to socialise with their peers and to learn about social norms (Berry and Dawkins 2004).

As well as having the right to education opportunities, in the UK it is recommended that wherever possible children with additional health or learning needs should be enabled to learn in a mainstream education environment. The caveats to this are unless their parents or guardians choose otherwise or this is 'incompatible with the efficient education of other children' and there are no 'reasonable steps' that the school and Local Education Authority can take to prevent that incompatibility (Ofsted 2004). The Disability Discrimination Act (HMSO 2005) places duties on schools to avoid treating disabled pupils less favourably than others and to make 'reasonable adjustments' to ensure that they are not disadvantaged. The Disability Discrimination Act applies to extracurricular as well as school-time activities, and means that children who have disabilities should be enabled to participate, if they wish to do so, in the range of activities associated with school life open to other children.

The benefits that inclusion in mainstream education offers, like inclusion in society as a whole, extend beyond the child or young person who has complex health needs. Their presence in mainstream schools gives their peers an opportunity to learn how to communicate with and include children and young people who have complex health needs, and to see them as people and as a part of mainstream society (Berry and Dawkins 2004). This could be seen as a fulfillment not only of the right of the child or young person who has complex health needs, but also of other children's right to education which prepares them for 'a responsible life in a free society, in the spirit of understanding, peace and tolerance' (Office of the United Nations High Commissioner for Human Rights 1989).

Inclusion of children with special health or educational needs in mainstream schools is advocated as the ideal. It is nonetheless important to stress that children and young people who have additional needs must be provided with the additional support they need to make mainstream education meaningful for them and genuinely inclusive (Russell 2003; Berry and Dawkins 2004). This means that they should be enabled to participate in classes with other children, and to be involved in all the activities they want, like any other child or young person. Inclusion is not achieved if a person who has additional needs attends a mainstream school but is unable to participate in activities with other pupils.

There are instances where children and young people who have complex health needs do not benefit from mainstream education. Berry and Dawkins

(2004) identify that poor understanding of their needs and abilities, or a lack of staff who can support them effectively means that they can be excluded from certain aspects of the curriculum in mainstream environments. If children with additional needs are obliged to spend the majority of the school day away from their peers, and have very limited opportunities to mix with them, their education is not truly inclusive. It may even detract from an inclusive ethos by marking them out as different and segregated (Hewitt-Taylor 2007).

Some mainstream schools are unable to provide for a child's medical needs. Children who have health related needs (such as tube feeding or the administration of medication during school hours) may be excluded from mainstream education because there are not enough staff who can perform these tasks, or because is a lack of clarity over who is responsible for them (Berry and Dawkins 2004). In some schools there is no one who is trained or prepared to give medication to pupils. This can mean that those who require medication during school hours are excluded from school altogether, or are obliged to leave classes and have their parents come into school to administer their medication (Berry and Dawkins 2004). This again sets them out as different from their peers, and means that they miss parts of lessons, which may not be easily caught up, particularly if this occurs regularly. This can mean that they do not have truly equal access to the amount of education compared with their peers.

As well as health related procedures being a potentially problematic area, Zijlstra and Vlaskamp (2005) found that school staff are not always clear about which situations or changes in health status merit a child missing lessons and which do not. They found that fairly minor issues such as drowsiness or increased temperature can mean that children and young people miss out on school activities or are sent home. This could sometimes be avoided if the staff were more aware of how their condition could be managed and learning still facilitated.

Sometimes children and young people who have complex health needs have a number of absences from school because of ill health. However, they may also miss considerable hours of school time because of the number of health related appointments that they have to attend (Department of Health 2004a). Enabling children to participate fully in education requires good communication between health, social care and education providers so that the child's needs are understood and met and their absences are minimised by effective planning of appointments. In some cases, funding and carer availability may need to be carefully considered so that children are offered education opportunities for longer than the usual number of school terms or the chance to catch up during holidays, to compensate for time that has been lost because of their health needs (Hewitt-Taylor 2007). This may be a move towards enabling children and young people who have complex health needs to have equal access to education in terms of hours actually spent in learning, not just time spent enrolled at a school or college.

Children with disabilities are often reliant on appropriate transport services to access education and a lack of suitable transport can preclude children attending the best school for them (Berry and Dawkins 2004). If they need, or may need, medication or treatment whilst they are on transport this has to be catered for in order for children and young people to access education (Berry and Dawkins 2004). Funding and practical arrangements for education therefore need to include resources, including appropriate transport and staff, to enable children and young people to travel safely to and from school or college.

Sometimes, where a child has specific medical or technical needs, a school which is used to providing the type of support that they need can more confidently include them in a range of activities (Hewitt-Taylor 2007). Thus, although inclusion is the aim, and the ideal, parents and their children also have a number of individual considerations to take into account when ascertaining which school or college is best for them, and what will give the child or young person the best opportunities and enable them to achieve what matters most to them.

Case study

Joanna attends mainstream school. She goes to the same lessons as her peers. The teachers and other pupils in her class have learned how her communication aid works and many have learned to lip-read her. She uses a combination of recording lessons, specialist computer equipment, her communication aid, her teachers lip-reading her, and her carer's co-operation to participate in classes and complete her course work.

Joanna's peers know that Joanna wants to be involved in the same activities as them, and many of them take great trouble to ensure that she can join in their break time activities, and get a chance to join in their discussions and be a part of the group.

When her class does sport, Joanna has the choice of watching, going for a walk with her carer or another agreed activity. Although she cannot be a part of a sports teams, she enjoys watching matches and often supports the school team at home matches. She cannot attend away matches and is limited in how many home matches she can go to because of the amount of support provided for her out of school hours.

Caroline explains how impressed she has been by Joanna's school: 'They are just a regular comprehensive school, but they have always had such a positive attitude. You know: "Well, let us know what's needed and what you want and what Joanna wants, and I'm sure we can sort something out." Nothing ever seems a big deal. They always just include her, like everyone else, and it was: "What do we need to put in place so that Joanna can do her GCSEs?" It wasn't: "can she?" or even: "We think maybe she can." It was "She's able to, so she is, and we just need to find out what do we need to do to get it organised so she gets the grades she deserves." I think because the Head Teacher has always been so positive, everyone else has just come on board.'

As well as having an adverse effect on children and young people, problems in them accessing education can affect their families. Their parents often have to be available during school hours in case their child is sent home, and may have to attend school themselves to assist with medical procedures (Berry and Dawkins 2004; Hewitt-Taylor 2007). This means that they may be unable to engage in paid employment, or commit to any other activities, as they cannot rely on being available because of their child's needs and the lack of provision for these.

THE RIGHT TO PRIVACY

The United Nations Convention on the Rights of the Child (Article 16) states that 'No child shall be subjected to arbitrary or unlawful interference with his or her privacy, family, home or correspondence, nor to unlawful attacks on his or her honour and reputation' (Office of the United Nations High Commissioner for Human Rights 1989). In healthcare, respect for privacy and confidentiality is an ethical and legal obligation (McLelland 2006). Confidentiality and privacy are discussed in more detail in relation to supporting children and their families at home in Chapter 5, and in relation to ethics in Chapter 9. However, children and young people have a right to privacy, and healthcare staff are required to respect their privacy.

Privacy includes physical privacy, privacy of thoughts, feelings, emotions and privacy in communication with others. Children and young people who have complex health needs have the same rights as other children and young people in this respect, and the staff who work with them have an obligation to respect their privacy. However, they may find achieving privacy very difficult. In many cases, they require a carer or other adult with them all the time, and every response they make, feeling they express, gesture or activity is open to observation by another person. Their private 'space', such as their room and home, may, of necessity, be seen and intruded upon on a regular basis by their family and carers. Their choices of environment, clothing and activities may be more closely observed or commented on than those of their peers. The nature of the care they need may require disclosure and discussion of the most personal details of their life and reveal very private facts about their body (Olsen et al. 2005).

Thus, a child or young person who has complex health needs is almost certain to be subject to limitations on their privacy in comparison to their peers. Supporting them effectively includes considering ways in which this can be reduced to the absolute minimum and sensitivity and respect for confidentiality in handling private information and intimate knowledge of them and their lives.

DEVELOPING INDEPENDENCE

Independence can be defined as: 'freedom from outside control or influence' (Soanes et al. 2001). This contrasts with dependence, which has been defined as 'reliance on someone or something' or 'unable to do without someone or something' (Soanes et al. 2001). Independence includes physical, social, emotional and intellectual elements and being independent contributes to the development of positive self-esteem. Children and young people who have complex health needs, like other children, need the opportunity to become independent. However, they may have more limitations on their independence and the development thereof than other children or young people. This is discussed in more detail in relation to the transition to adulthood in Chapter 6. However, the principle applies to children and young people of all ages.

Children who have complex health needs may be physically unable to be completely independent, for example they may require assistance with physical tasks, transport, communication, correspondence, and to access play and leisure activities. However, this should not be confused with their right or ability to engage in independent decision making, and the development of emotional and psychological independence.

More problematic than the need for physical assistance may be other people's attitudes impairing the development of independence in children and young people who have complex health needs. They, like other children, need to be allowed to make their own choices, to express themselves, and make their preferences known. Opportunities for a child or young person with complex health needs to develop their maximum level of independence in every area should be a goal, whatever their age, so that this process is a natural continuation at adolescence, rather than a new idea or task.

Case study

Andrew likes to choose what clothes he wears, and his parents almost always let him do this. They take him shopping for his clothes and he selects what he likes, and then chooses what he will wear every day. They also encourage him to tell them what he would like to do, and, when this is not possible, they discuss this with him and explain why. Paula explains that: 'There are so many things Andrew can't do, but he knows what he wants, and I like to let him choose as often as possible. Partly because, why shouldn't he, but also because if he gets used to that now, he will know he has the right to stand up for himself, to say what he wants in life, even in small things like what he wants to wear. I will always fight for him, but if anything happens to me or his Dad, I want him to know that he can choose, and he can tell people what he wants. It doesn't mean he always gets what he wants. I have three children, so if they all want different things on TV, or to go to a different place, then they can't all choose. They have to take turns. He has to learn that too. That side of things, the limits on choices, can be hard too though, because often there's a limit anyway to where we can go with Andrew, because of his wheelchair, but as much as possible, they all take it in turns to choose, like other siblings would.'

SUMMARY

Children and young people who have complex and continuing health needs have the same rights and needs as any other child or young person, in addition to their specific health related needs. The support they are provided with should focus on meeting their needs as children or young people, and as a part of a family, not just on their medical or technical needs. This involves ascertaining what is most important for them, and what they see as important in achieving quality of life on a day-to-day and longer term basis. Good communication is essential in ascertaining a child or young person's priorities, values and aspirations. The importance of the support which is provided in maximising the opportunities children and young people have to communicate, and to develop their skills and confidence in this, cannot be overstated.

Children and young people who have complex health needs have the right to participate in and enjoy play activities and leisure pursuits, and to spend time with their peers. They also have the right to the opportunity to engage in education, and should be enabled to develop their maximum level of independence in the same way that other children and young people do. The support they are provided with should have the aim of facilitating this. They also have the right to privacy, and the support they receive should be sensitive to this right.

Chapter 3
The Child or Young Person as a Part of the Family

The families of children and young people are usually a very significant part of their lives, and can be even more important when they have complex health needs. As Chapter 2 identifies, children and young people who have complex health needs often have less opportunities than their peers to spend time with other people; their families therefore form a very important part of their social world. In addition, they often depend on their families for a great deal of their daily care and support.

As well as their family being an important part of their lives, the needs of a child or young person who has complex and continuing health needs can impact on the whole family. The providers of support for these children and young people should therefore consider them not only as individuals, but as a part of their family. It should be planned to maximise quality of life for the family as a whole and to enhance the child or young person's ability to be and feel a part of, not just live in the same house as, their family.

FAMILY

A part of providing effective support to children, young people and their families is understanding what the term family means for those concerned. A family has been described as 'a group consisting of parents and their children living together as a unit, a group of people related by blood or marriage, the children of a person or couple, all the descendants of a common ancestor' (Soanes et al. 2001). However, what is seen as a family, the structure of what are considered to be families, how family members are regarded and expected to be involved with one another, and the norms related to families and family life varies between individuals, cultures and societies.

Two phrases that have been commonly used to describe families in western culture are the 'nuclear family' (used to describe a family group consisting of parents and their children) and the 'extended family' (which refers to a network of relatives that extends beyond the nuclear family) (*Encyclopaedia Britannica* 2006). However, there have been considerable changes in how families are organised, viewed, and in their function in western society over the twentieth century. This has inlcuded a trend away from people living and functioning as extended families to the nuclear family being the more common functional family unit. More recently, the nuclear family has ceased to be the dominant type of family, and a wide variety of relationships and groupings of people have become accepted structures for a family. These include: blended families, single-parent families and couples who do not have children. As a result, there is no longer, in many western societies, a typical family structure. In addition, although familial relationships are often described in genetic terms, the term 'family' may include people who are important to, close to, and involved in the upbringing of a child, despite having no genetic or legal relationship to them.

In the same way that family structures have changed over the years, so too have the economic functions of the family. It is possible that the family in a traditional western society formed the primary economic unit, however, this role has gradually diminished with the increasingly varied structure and function of families, and changes in division of labour within families. The economic function of a family, like its structure, is now highly individualised and variable.

Staff who work with children and young people who have complex health needs and their families should respect the way in which each family is structured and functions, their strengths and limitations, beliefs and values. The child or young person's family, whatever this means to them, is a constant in their life, whereas service providers are visitors (Samwell 2005). Working effectively with children, young people and their families requires staff to establish who the individuals concerned see as their family, who has parental responsibility for the child or young person with whom they work, who those with parental responsibility want involved in their lives and that of their child, who has a right of access to the child and in what circumstances, and who is important to and able to assist the child or young person and their parents.

PARENTING

The reason why an individual has parental responsibility for a child, and the way in which they view and carry out their parenting role is likely to be as varied as family structure. The term 'parent' means different things in different situations and to different individuals (Gage et al. 2006). A parent is defined as 'a mother or father' (Soanes et al. 2001). This can include being a biological parent, an adoptive parent, a foster parent or step parent (Soanes et al. 2001). Likewise, the routes taken to parenthood include being a child's biological parents, adoptive parents, foster parents, and step parents. A child may therefore have more than two persons who act in a parenting role, for example, a biological mother and father and an adoptive mother and father.

For those supporting families, it is important to be aware of all those who have parental claims on the child, how these claims affect their rights and the rights of the child, who has parental responsibility for the child, who should be involved in decision making regarding the child, and whose views should hold greatest strength. The reasons why and circumstances in which individuals can hold parental responsibility for a child, and the implications of this, are described in the Children Act (Department of Health 2004b). However, as well as being aware of who has legal responsibility as a child's parent, it is also necessary for staff to be aware of who the child or young person sees as important, enjoys being with and having in their lives.

Whatever the route taken to becoming a parent, the transition to parenthood is an event that creates significant changes for those taking on the role, and for their families. Becoming a parent is a major life transition, and alters a person's personal and social identity. It requires them to take on new roles and responsibilities and to incorporate an extra person into any existing relationships (Gage et al. 2006). This may mean making adjustments to the roles that individuals take on within relationships, the priorities which they afford to other people and aspects of their lifestyle and activities. In addition to adjusting existing relationships, values and priorities, parents often have to reevaluate the priorities which they afford to everyday tasks, employment, leisure, and social activities (McCourt 2006).

McCourt (2006) identifies that, with some exceptions, women in western society generally continue to assume the role of primary carer for a new baby, usually almost immediately after the baby's birth. Although this is often described as a time of great happiness, the adaptation which it requires and the need to fulfill one's own and society's expectations and take on new responsibilities can be an overwhelming and isolating experience (George 2005). The romanticised images that surround the mothering role, suggesting that it is instinctive and effortless, can add to the stress parents experience when this is not the case (McCourt 2006).

The way in which the role of mother is constructed in most modern post-industrialised societies makes great demands on women. The low status afforded to mothering and the suggestion that this is instinctive and almost effortless devalues the work of bringing up a child. This can have a negative impact on women's self-esteem when this is a major part of their life, particularly if they give up 'important' paid work to start their new 24-hour-a-day responsibility as a mother (McCourt 2006). At the same time, despite the lowly status afforded to being a parent, it is expected that parents will nurture their children and create an environment conducive to their social, emotional and cognitive development (Gage et al. 2006).

BEING THE PARENT OF A CHILD WHO HAS COMPLEX NEEDS

The transition to parenthood and the roles and responsibilities taken on by parents are potentially very challenging and time consuming, with little reward from society as a whole, despite children themselves being a source of considerable reward for many parents. When a child has complex and continuing health needs, taking on the role of being their parent presents additional challenges, both at the time of transition to parenthood and in the ongoing role of being their parent.

Parents whose child has complex needs have to manage all the usual aspects of the transition to parenthood, but as Phoenix et al. (1991:123) identify 'To be the mother of a disabled child is to be different.' Not only do their parents have to adjust to parenthood, they may have to adjust to being a different parent from what they and others had expected. Parents and other family members usually plan for the arrival of a new baby before they are born, consider the impact on themselves and their family and dream and think logically of what the future may hold for them. They therefore have to adapt these expectations when the processes they had anticipated do not take place, when their child is different from their expectations, and the outlook for them as parents changes (Barr and Millar 2003).

When it becomes evident during pregnancy, at, or around the time of their birth, that a baby will have ongoing health needs, their parents' expectations of their baby's birth and the time immediately after this may be changed. Their adaptation to their new role may be complicated by the environment in which they find themselves, and by the activities and nurturing which they were expecting to experience with their baby being changed.

When an older child develops a long-term health related condition or is involved in an incident that results in them developing complex and continuing health needs, the dreams, hopes and plans which their parents had developed for them over the years may have to change. Some specific aspects of this are discussed in more detail in Chapter 7, in relation to loss. However, what it means to be a parent, and what individuals and families will do and how they will be seen as parents are likely to change when a child has or develops complex and continuing health needs.

All parents have to develop a relationship with their child. However, this can be more difficult for parents whose child has complex needs than for other parents. They may be separated from their baby soon after their birth, sometimes by many miles if the baby needs specialist care or local neonatal cots are not available. They may be unable to hold their newborn baby as they expected, and may have to divide their time between other children at home and the newborn baby in hospital. This may mean that their early communication with their baby is not established in the way that it would be in other situations. Where a baby remains in hospital for some time, their parents cannot always be with them as much as they would otherwise be and have to develop their relationship with them in a very public environment. When a child develops complex health needs later in their childhood, parents may have to adapt their relationship with their child and expectations of this, again possibly at a distance from home and in a strange environment with very limited privacy.

Where a newborn baby who has additional health needs has siblings, their initial relationship with their brother or sister is unlikely to be as they expected, and the way in which the new baby integrates with the whole family is likely to be changed. When an older child develops complex health needs, their siblings also have to adjust to the changes in their brother or sister, and how this affects them, their lives, and their family as a whole.

Case study

Katrina was born at 26 weeks gestation. She spent her first 18 months of life in hospital. It was, for many weeks, uncertain whether or not she would survive. She required assisted ventilation for three months.

Katrina's parents, Nicola and Gary, spent the first weeks of their baby daughter's life in and around the neonatal intensive care unit. They were seldom able to hold her, and when they could, a member of staff was always with them. When she was uncomfortable, her position was changed, or her pain relief increased, but they could not spontaneously pick her up and cuddle her to comfort her.

Katrina was fed via a nasogastric tube, rather than being breastfed as Nicola had planned. Nicola or Gary sometimes held the syringe which was used to feed her if they were present for her feeds. They could not dress her in the clothes they had purchased. They could not take her home to the room which they had prepared. She never slept in the Moses basket which they had bought. Instead, they lived at the hospital with short visits home for the first 18 months of her life and Katrina slept in an incubator, then a bassinet, then finally a large hospital cot. When Nicola brought Katrina's own linen in, it was often lost amidst the hospital laundry. The same happened with a lot of her clothes. Nicola explains: 'I know it's a small thing, when she had so much being done for her, but we had chosen the first clothes she could wear and sheets and a blanket for her, and they all got lost. So, I don't have those that I can keep. It was one way we could make her ours. Make things a tiny bit as we had planned, and it just got lost. It's a very small thing, I know, but, for us, it did matter.'

Nicola and Gary's first weeks as parents were full of anxiety, and friends contacted them to express concern and sympathy, not congratulations on Katrina's birth. Katrina's first weeks of life included discussion of whether to continue treatment and what her short- and long-term prospects of survival and quality of life were. No one celebrated her arrival.

As they grow older, children who have complex health needs will often require their parents to care for them for longer, and with more intensity, than other children. Their needs may become more demanding as they become older and physically heavier to care for, and when the education opportunities and social activities, which are sometimes available to them through school, diminish. This may be a time at which other parents are considering their child leaving home and having more time to themselves to develop personal interests or careers (Todd and Jones 2005).

Although for many parents whose children have complex and continuing health needs the long-term nature of their responsibility is demanding and exhausting, it can also be very rewarding. However, Todd and Jones (2005) report that even the rewards which parents can derive from caring for their child may be tainted by others judging them harshly for expressing this. This can mean that, whatever the challenges and rewards which they experience, mothers and fathers whose children have complex health needs can feel marginalised, unsupported and devalued in their role as their child's parents.

As well as the changes in their expectations of parenthood, parents whose children have complex health needs have to contend with society's perceptions of and responses to them and their child. Phoenix et al. (1991:123) identifies that from the time of their baby's birth, a mother who has a disabled child is confronted by efforts being made to alter them, rather than to admire them and celebrate their arrival. Parents, whose baby is unwell or thought to be disabled, frequently do not receive the usual cultural markers acknowledging their baby's birth. Cards and celebrations may be withheld and embarrassment, silence and commiserations replace these. In some cases parents have to contend with hurtful and dismissive comments about their baby, or questions being asked by friends and relations regarding the worth of their survival (Green 2002; Hewitt-Taylor 2007).

Parents whose children have complex health needs may have to continue to contend with negative or unhelpful reactions to their child throughout their life, including their life being devalued by others (Kirk and Glendinning 2004; Carnevale et al. 2006). They may have to include in their protective role as parents protecting their child from hostile and unappreciative responses and debates over the value of their child's life. They not only have to define their child's talents and strengths, but to justify their child's worth and right to life in a way that other parents do not (Landsman 1998:78). This may mean that parents have to actively cognitively challenge and redefine the existing cultural understanding of what constitutes normality and perfection and review the way in which life and life's events are valued and measured by themselves and by society in a way that other parents do not (Landsman 2005; Fisher and Goodley 2007). Whilst this may enable them to achieve personal growth, and become more open minded, it is a task that other parents do not have to achieve as a part of being their child's parent. It can also mean that parents feel isolated from and unsupported by other parents, not because of their child, or their role as their parents, but because of the way in which other people respond to their child, and to them as their parents (Landsman 2005). As well as altering their experience of being a parent, the differences in how they perceive their child and themselves, and how society sees and values them can discourage parents from going out with their child into what can be a hostile environment. This can mean that they feel and become socially isolated and unsupported.

EXPERT PARENTS

Parents whose children have complex and continuing health needs develop highly specialist skills and knowledge, which makes them uniquely able to care for their child. However, this can significantly alter the meaning of parenting for them and change their expected role as parents (Kirk et al. 2005). For example, oral feeding is considered an important part of babies bonding with their parents. Where this is not possible, or difficult, an early and important act of parenting, to which many women attach great significance, may be lost, modified, or become a source of struggle rather than an opportunity for developing a close relationship with their baby. If a child is unable to feed orally and requires assisted feeding, one of their parents' expected nurturing roles may instead become a clinical procedure (Hazel 2006).

As well as the changes in their expected parenting role, parents whose children have complex health needs usually have to take on additional practical roles and responsibilities (Kirk and Glendinning 2004). These include gaining knowledge and practical skills related to their child's condition and taking on responsibility for medical and technical aspects of their child's care, roles which are closer to that of healthcare professionals than the expected roles of parents (Abbott et al. 2005; Kirk et al. 2005). One specific aspect of parenting that changes when parents have to provide medical or technical care for their child is having to perform clinical procedures on them to maintain their health. Whilst this is essential for their child's well-being, carrying out such procedures may be distressing for parents because they often involve deliberately inflicting pain or discomfort on their child rather than protecting them from suffering (Kirk et al. 2005).

As well as the usual decisions that parents have to make about their child, parents whose children have complex health needs have to develop highly specialised observation and decision-making skills related to their child's state of health, often noting very subtle but vital clues, acting on these and managing the fine tuning of the interventions and care which they need (Kirk et al. 2005). Parents also become involved in organising services and advocating for their child in a more intense and long-term way than other parents have to (Kirk and Glendinning 2004).

Whilst these roles and responsibilities mean that parents have very specialist knowledge of their child and their needs, they can also mean that they experience role ambiguity and conflict (Abbott et al. 2005; Kirk et al. 2005; Wang and Barnard 2004). They may at times feel, and be regarded by others, including healthcare professionals, more as nurses than as parents. Although they are often regarded by other parents and professionals as highly specialist and dedicated parents, Kirk et al. (2005) found that parents whose children have complex health needs generally want to be seen primarily as their child's parents, not defined by the health related activities that they undertake for their child. In addition, their attachment to and feelings for their child are those of a parent, not a professional.

Parenting in society is generally devalued (Green 2002; Scorgie and Sobsey 2006). Where a child has complex health needs, the absolute involvement that parents have in being the parents and the energy they expend on this is not always valued by society. When taken alongside the tendency of society to devalue the child to whom they devote extraordinary care and attention this may, unsurprisingly, have a negative impact on the parents' self-esteem and perception of their own as well as their child's perceived worth within society. This can mean that they not only have to fight to demonstrate their child's worth, but also their own worth as a parent and the value of the activities which can, quite literally, take over their whole life (Hewitt-Taylor 2007).

Case study

Katrina is now three. She requires oxygen (via nasal cannulae) 24 hours a day. Nicola has to make sure that this and her oxygen saturation monitor are in place all the time, that both are working correctly, and has to respond to any alarms, identify the cause of any problems, and decide what to do about these. If Katrina has a chest infection, Nicola often has to perform suction on her. Katrina is fed via a nasogastric tube, and Nicola gives her feeds, and replaces the nasogastric tube when necessary. Katrina is booked to have a gastrostomy performed, so Nicola is preparing to learn about caring for her gastrostomy and gastrostomy feeding. She also organises Katrina's appointments, and makes sure she has all the supplies which she needs, alongside meeting all the usual needs of a toddler, but with the additional considerations that Katrina has very limited mobility and is still in nappies. When they go out, she has to take Katrina, and all the necessary equipment, including an oxygen cylinder, spare oxygen cylinder, any feeds she will need, equipment to test the nasogastric tube position and administer the feed, supplies such as nappies and wipes, and things to entertain Katrina if they are out for long.

Nicola worked as a manager of a branch of a bank before she had Katrina, and had planned to return to work full time. Instead, she has taken a five-year career break, to see 'how things work out'. She describes how her previous colleagues veer between admiration ('You are amazing to do all this') and dismissing her role ('Aren't you bored just being at home. Can't they send someone in so you could come back to work, even just for a couple of days?') She explains how: 'I want to be with Katrina. It is more rewarding than anything else I have ever done, she is my little girl, and I love her. I don't want people to think I am a hero just because I look after her, but at the end of the day, I do a lot, and if I didn't, it would cost thousands of pounds for someone else to look after her. So yes, I do want to do it, and I don't want to make a fuss, but, no I'm not bored, I don't have time to be bored, and I probably do things and make decisions which are more complicated than any of them do. It's not just that. We don't know how things will turn out for Katrina. I don't know how long I've got her for, and much as some people have spelled that out to me, said I have to have a life in case anything happens to her, equally, because I don't know how long I have with her, I don't want to be sorting out someone else's bank account when I could be with her.'

THE IMPACT OF HAVING A CHILD WHO HAS COMPLEX NEEDS

Whilst much of the literature on being the parent of a child who has complex and continuing health needs emphasises the stressors of this role, it is also important to describe the rewards and enrichment which the child itself brings to their parents and family (Redmond and Richardson 2003). In general, the stressors related to having a child who has complex health needs are a result of the demands imposed by the practicalities of the care they need, the social barriers their parents encounter and the stigma society creates, not the child itself (Green 2007). Kearney and Griffin (2001) describe the love and hope that parents experience with their child, and Landsman (2005) identifies that the majority of mothers whose children have complex health needs grow to value their child's positive attributes, qualities, and quality of life.

As well as the pleasure that a parent whose child has complex health needs has in their child as a person, and their relationship with them, Lassetter et al. (2007) describe how some parents find that their experiences with their child make them more aware of others and their needs. Many mothers report that being their child's parent enables them to achieve personal growth and to prioritise their lives, discard outdated beliefs, learn new and positive values and to redefine what personal fulfillment means (Scorgie and Sobsey 2006; Green 2002; Wolfson 2004).

Despite the rewards which a child who has complex health needs may bring to their parents, for many parents theirs is a stressful role. The level of care which some children require means that their parents have an un-usually high level of responsibility and are subject to considerable physical demands and time management challenges (Heaton et al. 2005; Levine 2005). This includes the workload of moving and handling their child and any equipment they use, and assisting their child with eating, washing, dressing and toileting (Wang and Barnard 2004; Shribman 2007). These commitments, and the level of them, continue for much longer than would be the case for another child.

Although parents frequently provide care and interventions which would generally be the remit of professional staff as well as the usual parenting roles, they have no time 'off duty' from the physical care and constant vigilant watch-ing that their child needs (Abbott et al. 2005; Kirk et al. 2005). Many parents experience long-term sleep deprivation, due to the high level of vigilance re-quired 24-hours a day and the noise of machinery or alarms at night, which may be disruptive even when another person is employed to care for their child (Wang and Barnard 2004). This level of responsibility and the extraordi-nary level of care and attention that parents must devote to their child's needs can be overwhelming and become their entire life (Kirk et al. 2005; Carnevale et al. 2006).

Parents often feel that they have no choice in taking on the extremely de-manding role and workload which their child's health needs occasion. Their desire to have their child living at home often means that they accept, by default, the responsibility for the constant monitoring that their child re-quires and carrying out a range of clinical and care related procedures (Kirk et al. 2005). Their willingness to undertake these tasks is reinforced by the expectation that a parent will take on responsibility for whatever care their child needs (Judson 2004). As has already been identified, this expectation often contrasts with the value that society subsequently places on the role which parents in general and particularly those whose children have complex health needs take on.

As well as meeting their child's direct care needs, parents often spend a great deal of time and experience considerable stress from having to organise the support and services which they and their child need (Kirk et al. 2005; Buelow et al. 2006). This includes organising and coordinating services, and ensuring that they had sufficient supplies to care for their child. The organisation and administration involved in ensuring adequate support for their child, alongside all the other aspects of family life which parents have to deal with means that each day can feel like 'one endless battle' (Contact a Family 2004a).

Unsurprisingly, given their unrelenting and constant physical and emotional workload which they take on, parents whose children have complex health needs can themselves experience health problems associated with their role as carers. These include physical problems, such as back and joint pain from lifting and handling, and problems with their mental health and wellbeing (Contact a Family 2004a; Wang and Barnard 2004).

Many parents whose children have complex health needs have to live with a considerable degree of uncertainty (Levine 2005; Meehan 2005). This includes uncertainty over the child's health (Buelow et al. 2006; Wang and Barnard 2004), and awareness of the frailty of their child's life (Redmond and Richardson 2003; Judson 2004; Carnevale et al. 2006). Redmond and Richardson (2003) describe how, given the uncertainty of their child's prognosis, parents have to develop ways of dealing with this, often very pragmatically by living day to day, rather than making long-term plans. This makes their lives and outlook very different from that of other parents, who can plan further ahead for their children and families. It is also something which those providing support should take into account, because the way in which parents view their situation can appear to be at odds with that of professionals, when the reality may be that they are working in different time frames and with different values and priorities.

This combination of emotional and physical stress, with enrichment and pleasure, described by Meehan (2005) as 'joy and sorrow' is one which parents learn to live with. It is also one which service providers need to appreciate in order to provide effective support that enables parents to enjoy the positive aspects of being their child's parent, and their relationship with them, but reduce the stressors, including those associated with their child being devalued as a person.

Case study

George suffered a brain injury at birth. He is now fed via a gastrostomy, has difficulty communicating, cannot move independently, and is blind. His mother, Debra, cares for him, with some assistance financed by legal action for medical negligence. His father left the relationship when George was 17 months old.

George is now 16. It has been suggested to Debra that she consider George going to live in a residential setting, or another form of supported accommodation, or convert her house so that he can have 24-hour care independently of her and she can: 'get my life back'. However, she does not wish to do this. She wants to continue to care for her son, because 'He is my life now. He has been for 16 years.' Although she realises that other people: 'Think that it is odd, they wonder why I don't jump at the chance to do that. Other people just see his disabilities. They don't see him as a person. He has a fantastic sense of humour, and he is so loving. When I have a bad day, he always has a hug for me. I know what he needs, I know when he is happy, or sad. I know it takes all my day looking after him, and talking to social services, the nurses, sorting out the things he needs, his wheelchair, his feeds, his splints, his hoist, but he is my son. I couldn't leave him in a strange house, with people he doesn't know. Or move him into some annexe of this house and change his relationship with me. He wouldn't understand why. He has been here with me since he was a baby. We have never been apart. I have help with him, carers who help me with lifting, and take him out so I can do things on my own now and then. He is also at school all day and we are looking at college options. You know, other people work as nurses their whole lives. It's sometimes quite strange, the way people look at me when I say I like looking after him, as if my job looking after him is ... not just less important but something that it's odd I should want to do. No one thinks it odd that someone else would want to do it. A nurse who is nothing to him can work with him all her life, but when I, as his mother do, it's ... no one says it, but it is definitely seen as odd by some people.'

SOCIAL OPPORTUNITIES

The demands placed on parents whose children have complex health needs often mean that whilst they have very little time to themselves, they can also experience social isolation (Levine 2005). They may have difficulty in maintaining friendships because of the amount of things they have to juggle related to their child's care, and because outings having to be planned around the child's care needs and routines (Yantzi et al. 2006). Collecting and packing the equipment, medication, and feeds that their child will need whilst they are out and the physical energy required to get them ready, transfer them to and from a vehicle, and locate a venue where they can meet friends and bring their child can make socialising more of a difficulty than a pleasure. Some parents find going out almost impossible because the exhaustion and sleep deprivation which their child's needs cause them leaves them with insufficient reserves to plan and execute outings (Yantzi et al. 2006). Although having staff to assist in their child's care may reduce parents' workload, the presence of care staff in their home may also impinge on their social life if they feel disinclined to entertain friends with another person present (Kirk et al. 2005). This combination of factors can mean that parents whose children have complex health needs have very limited options for maintaining friendships and keeping in touch with relatives.

As well as the practicalities and time factors involved in maintaining friendships, parents may find that they lose common ground or experience with friends. Friends' responses to their child, and failure to understand the demands and rewards of their role, may also make it difficult to sustain existing relationships.

Case study

Debra has found, over the years since George was born, that she has lost contact with a number of friends and relations. Some of these were a result of the ending of her relationship with George's father, but in other cases, she recalls:

'When George was a baby, although things were very different for me than they were for my friends, he was still a baby, still needed much the same care as other babies. I could still take him out like my friends could. We could all go to the same places. I already felt a bit left out because I knew that George would never do a lot of the things they were planning for and discussing, but I could still join in. As he got older, and became noticeably different, people started to be less interested in him, and I stopped being able to do things with them and their children. Everything that he needs means we can't get out very early or easily, and a lot of the places my friends took their children to, he couldn't go. Then a lot of people didn't really want to hear about him. They wanted to talk about what their children were doing, but he was like ... it didn't matter what he was doing. They would talk about how hard it must be for me, but when that finished, they talked about their lives, their children. George never got a mention, except as a burden on me. If I ever mentioned what he was doing, it didn't fit the conversation really. It was just awkward. Their lives were so different that we lost touch over time, and now, I suppose I only really have a couple of friends.'

EMPLOYMENT AND FINANCES

Having a child who has complex health needs can significantly impact on their parents' employment opportunities and status. Mothers whose children have disabilities are much less likely to be in paid employment than other mothers. Only 16% of mothers with disabled children are employed, compared with 61% of other mothers (Department of Health 2004a; Brazier 2006). Donovan et al. (2005) found that many mothers whose children have disabilities would like to have more opportunities for employment and to be involved in activities outside their role as their child's parent. However, in most cases they cannot achieve this and the expectation is that they will give up or significantly modify their employment in order to care for their child (Judson 2004). A number of barriers, which parents, and in particular mothers, face when seeking to return to work, has been identified. These include: a lack of childcare which caters for children with additional needs; a lack of suitable care for disabled children in school holidays and after school; the need for parents to take time off work on a frequent and often unpredictable basis for hospital visits and appointments and when their child is not well enough to attend school; a lack of understanding and flexibility by employers regarding the child's needs and that these will not lessen over time. Fathers' employment and earnings are also often reduced compared with those whose children do not have disabilities (Contact a Family 2004a; Department of Health 2004a). The United Nations Convention on Rights of the Child (Article 18) states that: 'children of working parents have the right to benefit from child-care services and facilities for which they are eligible' (Office of the United Nations High Commissioner for Human Rights 1989). However, it seems that childcare opportunities and facilities for children who have disabilities are not equal to those children who are not disabled. This may be even more so when a child has complex and continuing health needs.

Changes in parents' employment can have a significant financial effect on their family. Although parents may receive state benefits for their role in their child's care, in many cases these will not be equivalent to their previous salary, or compensate for their salary losses (Abbott et al. 2005). In addition, parents commonly report difficulties in finding out about and claiming benefits and often find that very little assistance with financial management is available to them (Department of Health 2004a; Abbot et al. 2005).

At the same time as having reduced earnings because of their child's needs, the cost of bringing up a child who is disabled is significantly higher than the cost of bringing up another child (Department of Health 2004a). This includes the cost of housing adaptations, specialist furniture, toys and the cost of incidental expenses such as transport and electricity. (Hewitt-Taylor 2007). Thus, families who have a child who has complex and continuing health needs often have a reduced income whilst their outgoing expenses are increased (Department of Health 2004a). Unsurprisingly, financial concerns are common amongst parents whose children have complex health needs and can contribute significantly to the stress which families experience (Hewitt-Taylor 2007).

Changes in their employment status may also impact on parents' sense of personal identity, for example, if their career pathway is unexpectedly terminated or their role at work ceases to exist. Employment may enable some parents to have a sense of identity other than as their child's parent, which is important to them and which is lost if they are unable to work (Todd and Jones 2005). Changes in employment may also alter parents' opportunities for social interaction and for some parents going to work forms a break from the care routine which the child's needs impose. A lack of opportunity to be in paid employment means that they do not have this break from the practical demands of caring for their child (Yantzi et al. 2006). The employment changes which parents may experience as a result of their child's needs can therefore affect their sense of identity and well-being.

It is acknowledged that parents whose children have complex needs develop very specialist knowledge and skills which exceed those of many professionals (Kirk and Glendinning 2004; Kirk et al. 2005). This nonetheless receives relatively little recognition in society. This, added to the low status which mothering is generally afforded in society (McCourt 2006) may do little for the self-esteem of parents who change their employment status in order to support their child. This may not be because of their own perception of their worth, or the worth of the work of caring for their child, but because of how society sees and values them and their work. As well as parents whose children have complex health needs being enabled to have more opportunities to engage in paid employment, the value of their work as their child's parent requires greater recognition.

RELATIONSHIPS BETWEEN PARENTS

Having a child who has complex and continuing health needs can bring a couple closer together, but the additional pressures of looking after their child can also put considerable strain on a relationship (Contact a Family 2004b). Kirk and Glendinning (2004) identify that it can be difficult for parents to have a break from care and enjoy time together, because the usual range of babysitters, such as family and friends cannot cope with their child's needs and it is sometimes not appropriate that they should do so unless they have received specialised training. In addition, the roles which parents take on in their relationship and in relation to their child may be very different, for example if one partner continues to engage in paid work whilst the other cares for the child. This may mean that they lose common ground, or resent the role which the other takes on and that the effects of their child's needs are very different for each of them. The level of exhaustion and loss of sleep that many parents experience may be detrimental to relationships as may stressors over the organisational aspects of their child's care, and financial concerns (Hewitt-Taylor 2007). Parents may also have different views on and responses to their child's needs, how these should be catered for, and different ways of coping with the demands which their child's needs bring (Hewitt-Taylor 2007).

EFFECTS ON THE FAMILY

A child having complex and continuing health needs can impact on their whole family. Carnevale et al. (2006) and Levine (2005) found that families whose children have complex health needs make great efforts to develop routines which enable them to resemble other families and to create a stable family life and home environment. However, there are still many factors that disrupt their lives and over which they do not have complete control (Wang and Barnard 2004).

For many families, having a child who has complex health needs changes their home and what home means to them (Wang and Barnard 2004). This can be because of the ingress of medical equipment, staff and professional visitors into their home, and can mean that what was the family's personal space is no longer their own (Kirk and Glendinning 2004; Wang and Barnard 2004). Although support can be vital for families, the number of individuals and services involved in their lives can leave them feeling overwhelmed by visitors. This can impinge on their time to enjoy family activities, and can constitute a considerable intrusion on their privacy (Glendinning and Kirk 2000; Wang and Barnard 2004). The presence of staff in the family home can mean that the family's lives are conducted alongside staff who are comparative strangers, and that their interactions, emotions, behaviours, and lifestyles are open to public inspection and judgement (Brett 2004; Kirk et al. 2005).

Whilst living in suitable housing and having appropriate equipment and assistive technology are often important to meet a child or young person's health needs, they may also disrupt the family's home. For example, finding space to store equipment and supplies may be difficult, and may mean that the family home needs to be adapted, or that the family have to relocate to a more suitable property (Abbott et al. 2005). This constitutes a disruption to the existing family situation and may mean that the family's house is no longer the home they chose, or wanted (Hewitt-Taylor 2007).

When a child or young person has complex health needs, their family's life often revolves around the routines and constraints that their needs impose (Kirk and Glendinning 2004). In the same way that organising going out with their child may make social activities difficult for parents, it may make family outings problematic (Kirk and Glendinning 2004; Abbott et al. 2005). Staff visiting the home, or the child or young person having to attend appointments, can interrupt the family's everyday activities and mean that events and outings have to be planned around these (Glendinning and Kirk 2000; Wang and Barnard 2004). This means that day-to-day events that other families might take for granted, such as taking the child's siblings to and from school and out of school activities, require considerable planning and may even become impossible (Kirk and Glendinning 2004).

When parents can organise days out for the whole family, they often have problems finding locations that will be suitable for all their children and facilities which all the family can enjoy (Rehm and Bradley 2005). Rehm and Bradley (2005) identify that when a venue is unsuitable for the whole family or does not provide activities that everyone can enjoy, the family have to separate, and do not have the chance to be a 'family' in the way that other families do. Alternatively, they have to limit their activities to venues that cater for children who have complex health needs, which may mean that the child's siblings miss out on activities which they would enjoy. Days out may need to end earlier than would usually be the case because the child who has complex health needs has to come home to begin therapies, feeds, or to be in bed in time for therapies to be commenced or for staff to arrive (Kirk and Glendinning 2004).

If a family wants to go on holiday, this often requires many months of planning and organisation. Travelling abroad may be so difficult and costly that families do not attempt it (Glendinning and Kirk 2000). However, even within the United Kingdom, holidays can be very difficult to organise, and much more expensive than they are for other families. For example, special transport arrangements may need to be made, and if the family need care staff to accompany them, policy and practices vary regarding what costs will be met by NHS or Primary Care Trusts. In some cases families have to meet the cost of staff salaries, transport and accommodation, which makes even holidays within the UK very costly (Hewitt-Taylor 2007).

The locations that families can use for holidays and options for accommodation are often limited. The limitations that families face include considerations of access to and within the property, electricity supply, space for storage of equipment and supplies, and safety concerns.

The work of organising a holiday when it includes a child who has complex health needs involves ensuring that all the required supplies are available and can be transported to the holiday location. This often restricts where a family can go to and, where car hire is needed, the size of vehicle hired, and the cost. Holiday insurance is usually much higher for children who have complex health needs, and, if the family plan to travel abroad, may be prohibitive (Hewitt-Taylor 2007). This combination of factors means that some families consider holidays too difficult to contemplate, even within the UK (Abbott et al. 2005).

Case study

Teresa and Diego have three children. Alejandro, who is 8, Marcos, who is 5 and Alicia who is 3. Alicia needs oxygen at night, and is fed via a gastrostomy. She has very limited mobility. Teresa explains:

'Every day, I have to get up, get Alicia's feed done, then make sure the boys are ready for school. Then I have to get everyone in the car, and get them all to school. I still have to carry Alicia. I have to carry her to the car and put her in, and she is heavy now she is three. She is small for her age, but she is heavy to carry. Another three-year-old would walk to the car and just need to be lifted into the seat. So, Alejandro has to make sure Marcos is safe, and help him a bit.

'Then, if Alejandro has football, or anything else after school, I have to think about how I can do that. There are no nurseries here that will take Alicia, with her needs, so I have to go and collect Marcos at three, and maybe Alejandro an hour later. So, each time, like any other mother, I need to take all the children, but each time I have to carry Alicia to and from the car, and then get her into her buggy when we get to the school. My friend has her three-year-old daughter at nursery from 1 pm until 4 or 5 pm so she collects her on the way back from the last school run. But I can't do that. Sometimes, Alejandro's friend's Mum will bring him home, but I don't like to do that too often, because I can't offer to collect them both ever. There isn't room for an extra child in my car with everything I need for Alicia.

'If we want to go out for a day, to the beach maybe, I have to think how I will get Alicia across the sand. Her buggy is no good on the sand, but she can't walk. She can't sit very well, so I need something she can sit in on the beach. So I have to carry that too. If my husband is with me, he helps, but in the holidays, he is at work and the boys still need to go out. Even if we go to the park, I can take her buggy, but I have to think: should she sit there for hours while they play? So I have to take a seat for her, and have that with me if we want to stay for a while. I have to take something for her to do, which mostly means large things. The boys will take a football, and play with that, and on the swings and slides, but Alicia needs things to do.'

Teresa's mother lives in Madrid, and is not well enough to travel to England. The family has not been able to take Alicia to see her. Before Alicia was born the family went to see her every year. The boys have not seen their grandmother for the past three years and Alicia has never seen her.

THE IMPACT OF THE CHILD'S NEEDS ON THEIR SIBLINGS

Having a sibling who has complex health needs may have an effect on the child's brothers and sisters. In addition, concerns about their nondisabled children can add to parental stress (Taylor et al. 2001; Abbott et al. 2005). The needs of the siblings of children and young people who have complex health needs are not always well catered for (Abbott et al. 2005). However, ensuring their well-being should be seen as equally important as the well-being of their brother or sister.

Sibling relationships are extremely complex and variable, and the roles traditionally taken on and accepted by siblings vary between cultures (Sanders 2004). Sibling relationships in general tend to be a mixture of emotions (Contact a Family 2007). Studies about the siblings of disabled people have similarly tended to report a mixed experience (Dodd 2004). One study reports that the siblings of disabled children have the same but stronger feelings about their brother and sister, liking or disliking them as frequently but with more intensity than a matched group did their nondisabled brothers and sisters (Contact a Family 2007). Children are often very close to their disabled brother or sister, but the relationship can include some specific difficulties. As with parents though, many difficulties that these brothers or sisters experience relate more to society and the provision which is made for children with complex health needs than the child itself.

Some children resent the increased attention that their disabled sibling receives, and the limitations that their needs impose on family activities. Some experience disturbed sleep, feel tired at school, miss school, or find it hard to complete homework because of their sister or brother's needs (McClure 2005; Carnevale et al. 2006; Contact a Family 2007). Some children are teased or bullied at school because of their siblings, or are embarrassed by their brother or sister's behaviour in public (Contact a Family 2007). Having to, or feeling that they have to, put their sibling's needs first seems to predispose to early maturity in the brothers and sisters of children who are disabled, and parents may worry that their nondisabled children have to grow up too quickly. However, the positive aspect of this is that they are often described as very responsible and sensitive to the needs and feelings of others. In addition, many adults whose siblings are disabled say that their brother or sister has brought something special to their lives (Contact a Family 2007; Hewitt-Taylor 2007).

The effects of having a disabled sibling is affected by a number of things, including: the frequency with which their brother or sister needs intervention; their own self-esteem; how far they feel supported; whether they can discuss their feelings with anyone; their parent's awareness of their feelings; the effects which their sibling's needs has on overall family functioning; the degree of emotional distress that their parents experience; their relationships with adults other than their parents; and how far the family value their brother or sister as a person (Taylor et al. 2001; Sharpe and Rossiter 2002; Contact a Family 2007).

Case study

Alejandro does a lot to help his mother, because he can see that she is busy. He seems happy to help her, and is very close to her. However, Teresa explains:

'He comes in from school, and he has homework to do, and he asks me: "Mami, do you need me to do anything?" Usually I try to say no, because he has work to do, but he watches me, and he notices things and he finds ways to help me. He always loads our dishwasher, he always comes and sets the table. He always helps me. Last week one day he came home and said "Mami, I have no homework today, so I can help you." I said to him "Alejandro, you go outside and play football with Marcos. You have no homework so it is your playtime. So he went, he ran out and he was smiling, but first he asked me. That breaks my heart, that he is so good, but he is so responsible. At his age, he shouldn't have to think that way.

'Last week, Alejandro told me he didn't have football. But I found he should have been at football practice. He thought it was so much work for me to collect him, so he decided to miss it. He loves football, and that made me feel so sad, he is so grown up, he tries to look after me too, to make my life easier, and he never puts himself first. I told him, and his teacher: "Alejandro can do football. Don't let him say no."'

Sometimes children provide a substantial amount of care for their siblings and are described as young carers. In 2004, 2142 children were provided with a significant amount of care by their siblings (Dearden and Becker 2004). The roles that siblings may take on include practical tasks such as cooking, housekeeping, shopping; physical care such as lifting and assisting with care; providing emotional support; caring for other siblings; and interpreting (McClure 2005). The responsibilities that they take on have a range of effects and young carers span a spectrum from being well-adjusted and supported to overburdened (McClure 2005). There is a general consensus that more attention should be given to the needs of children who assist in any way in the care and support of disabled siblings (Heaton et al. 2003). If siblings are involved in caring for their brother or sister, they may be entitled to an assessment of their needs in their caring capacity.

The Children Act (Department of Health 2004b) states that:

> the needs of brothers and sisters (of disabled children) should not be overlooked and they should be provided for as part of a package of services for the child with a disability.

Service provision should, therefore, take into account the needs of the siblings of children who have complex and continuing health needs, as well as the child or young person themselves. Dodd (2004) also found that support form of a sibling group can be beneficial for the brothers and sisters of disabled children as it provides peer support, understanding and sharing of ideas. Those who work with children and young people who have complex health needs may be able to advise their siblings about the existence of such groups.

THE IMPACT OF THE CHILD'S NEEDS ON THE EXTENDED FAMILY

Having a disabled child has an effect on the whole family (Contact a Family 2005). The extent of the effect on individual family members will depend on the family structure and functions, and the personalities and circumstances of individuals, but often includes grandparents (Green 2001). Hall (2004) found that grandmothers of critically ill children often experience a 'double concern' that encompasses the well-being or both their child and grandchild. The same may apply to children who have complex and continuing health needs, with grandparents having long-term concerns for their child and grandchild. Grandparents, like parents, may have a very different role from that which they expected in relation to their grandchild. Like parents, they may have to deal with different responses to their grandchild than would otherwise be the case, and may encounter prejudice, negative responses and lack of appreciation of their grandchild from society, on a long-term basis.

Case study

When Katrina was born, Nicola's parents found it very difficult to know what to do when they visited her. They had no clear role, and, as the rule was that Katrina was not allowed to have more than two visitors at any one time, if they visited either Gary or Nicola had to leave. The hospital was a one-hour bus journey away from their home, and Katrina's grandmother does not drive.

Katrina's grandparents were not congratulated on their new arrival, but were greeted with expressions such as 'What a shame'. 'Do you think it will be worth it?' (treating Katrina intensively) and 'But what will she be like if she does survive this? It's going to be hard work for your daughter.'

Katrina's grandparents had expected to provide a great deal of her care when her mother returned to work. However, they do not feel confident in managing her needs, so they occasionally care for her for an hour or so to give Nicola a break, but not for whole days.

Similarly, other members of the extended family (for example aunts or uncles) who are close to the parents of a child who has complex health needs, or the child or young person themselves, may find that they have to deal with changes in their own expected role and manage the way in which society views and comments on the child and their parents. They too may have a double concern, for the child and their parents, and feel unsure of the best way to support them.

SUMMARY

A child or young person having complex and continuing health needs has the potential to impact on their whole family, and on every aspect of their lives. Supporting children, young people and their families requires staff to understand the way in which the family is structured, who is important to the child or young person, who has legal rights to be involved in their life, and to what extent. Supporting the child's parents may be enhanced by staff thinking about the way in which their child's needs may have affected their parent's expectations, and how society responds to them as individuals and as parents.

Those who support children and their families need to attempt to identify what matters most for the child or young person but also how the support that is provided can best meet the needs which the family have as a result of the child or young person's needs, whilst preserving the rights of all the children in the family. The support that is provided should have as its aim enabling parents and families to enjoy the rewards and pleasures which the child or young person who has complex health needs brings them, and reduce the stressors associated with their health needs.

Chapter 4
Working with Parents

Healthcare professionals who work in the community always have to develop acceptable working relationships with the families with whom they work. However, when this involves working in the family home on a regular basis, often for full shifts, the relationship can be very different from that which is needed in other situations. Working in this way can mean that the relationships which develop between staff and families are more akin to the usual working relationships encountered between colleagues.

This chapter discusses some of the specific issues involved in working with children or young people who have complex and continuing health needs and their parents on a long-term, day-to-day basis.

NEGOTIATION

The development of good working relationships between children and young people who have complex health needs, their families and professionals requires a great deal of negotiation. Negotiation can be defined as the reaching of agreement or compromise through discussion (Saones et al. 2001). The process of negotiation may be formal or informal. Where families work very closely with healthcare staff, there is likely to be a combination of formal negotiation where expectations and agreements are set out and documented, and informal and ongoing day-to-day negotiation regarding almost every aspect of their work and relationships. Negotiations between staff and families may have to include: the aspects of the child or young person's care and support which the family want to manage; those in which they want to take the lead but have assistance with, those in which they want healthcare staff to take the lead but wish to remain involved; and any areas for which they would prefer staff to take full responsibility (Kirk 2001). Where the day-to-day care of a child or young person is involved, agreement over the role which staff are to play in their life and that of their family as well as in providing for their healthcare needs also has to be reached. In addition, the way in which staff use the family home, the facilities available to them and what will constitute the 'house rules' requires negotiation.

Renegotiation of the roles taken on by and relationships between staff and families are often necessary as the child's condition and age change, and as their parents become more confident in their child's care. The process of negotiation may also change as families become more accustomed to their role and to working with healthcare staff. This can mean that, for staff and families, the process of working together requires ongoing, sometimes almost daily negotiation. This is often a very informal and subconscious process, but nonetheless a part of the work of supporting families whose children have complex health needs. When new staff are appointed, a significant part of the negotiation process has to begin again and new working relationships have to be established. If there is difficulty in retaining staff, or staff are appointed on a short-term basis, this ongoing process can be exhausting for families (Hewitt-Taylor 2007).

One dynamic in any negotiation process is the power relationship that exists between the negotiating parties. Despite the rhetoric of empowerment of service users, it is possible that healthcare providers and service users cannot enjoy totally equal relationships, as the nature of healthcare provision is not usually one of choice (Ronayne 2001). This applies very much to the support that children and young people with complex health needs and their families receive. The encounter is one of necessity, not choice, insofar as most families would not choose to have staff in their homes; it is their child's needs that make this a necessity (Hewitt-Taylor 2007). It is sometimes supposed that, by being in their own home, parents can negotiate on an equal footing with healthcare staff. However, whilst many parents find that their position is one of greater power than would be the case in a hospital environment, being assertive in negotiating with professionals is not easy for families, even at home (Kirk 2001). Families may not perceive themselves as being in a position of equal power to service providers. This does not only pertain to their perceived status, but to their state of need. If parents feel themselves to be in need of assistance, which another individual or organization can bestow or withhold, they may feel unable to assert their preferences and negotiate with staff, of whatever grade, for fear that what help they have, however flawed, will be lost. Equally, staff may feel intimidated by confident parents, particularly if they fear that their jobs are insecure. To assume that both parties are negotiating from an equal footing is therefore unrealistic.

Case study

Christine and Susan's 23-month-old son, Tom, has a tracheostomy and requires CPAP at night. He is fed via a gastrostomy, with the majority of his feed being given overnight. He has very limited mobility.

Susan and Christine both worked full time before Tom was born. Susan now works three days a week as a teacher. Christine works from home as an IT consultant. They had expected to be able to send Tom to nursery when he was two, however they have had to reorganise their plans, and have both changed their working arrangements to facilitate this. They have learned to carry out all of Tom's care, but need someone with him at night so that they can sleep, so as to be able to manage his care between them during the day. They therefore have a carer to be with Tom at night (from 10 pm until 7 am).

Christine and Susan find that most of the staff seem to very genuinely care about Tom, interact well with him, and respect their home. However, one person regularly arrives 10–15 minutes late for her shift, never washes up after her meal break, and often has loud telephone conversations during the night, which Christine and Susan can hear, despite their room being separated from Tom's by another room. This disturbs them and Tom. In one conversation they heard her saying: 'Well, they get night care. They only have to look after him in the day, like any other parent does. If they don't want to take the trouble of looking after a child they should have thought about that before having one.'

Susan and Christine have spoken to the carer about this, but to no avail. Susan wants to ask if this member of staff can be replaced, but Christine feels that they cannot complain, because they receive some assistance, this member of staff usually only does two nights a week, and there are no guarantees that someone else could be found. Tom was in hospital until he was 14 months old because staff had to be recruited and trained to provide them with support and she feels that 'something may be better than nothing.'

BUILDING RELATIONSHIPS

Staff who support children and young people who have complex health needs will often spend many hours with them and their parents in the family home. This requires them to be nonjudgemental of the values and beliefs which parents hold, and means that they have to develop, find or agree on a common value system within which to work.

Being nonjudgemental means that individuals and families should not be judged on the basis of a member of staff's personal standards or opinions. It does not mean that staff should be unaware of or deny the differences between them and the families with whom they work. Being nonjudgemental requires an active discernment of one's own opinions, values and beliefs and awareness of how these might inform one's behaviour. Furthermore, to achieve nonjudgmental behaviour an individual needs the ability to use this awareness to actively seek to avoid allowing their own opinions, values and beliefs to have a negative impact on the support they provide to others (Koh 1999).

Values can be defined as 'principles, standards or behaviours' or 'the regard that something is held to deserve, importance or worth' (Soanes et al. 2001). When staff work closely with parents and regularly provide a great deal of direct care for their child, the congruence of the values they and the child's parents hold is important. These can include the moral and ethical values that individuals hold, and the values which they attach to various aspects of life. Where staff are involved in caring for a child on a frequent basis, the values and beliefs that inform parents' childcare practices and the ability of staff to work within these are also crucial to developing a good working relationship and providing good quality support. It can be difficult for staff and parents to work closely when their values are at odds on important matters, and the effects of vastly differing values being enacted every day can be problematic for the child in terms of consistency of expectations, rules, norms and practices.

Whilst it is unlikely that many individuals will be of complete accord in relation to all aspects of childcare, finding a value system and childcare practices which each party agrees to abide by is important. As parents have responsibility for their child 24 hours a day, unless, as may happen in exceptional cases, these are not in the child's best interests, theirs are the values that should hold priority. The task of staff is to support families in caring for their child, not to impose their value systems on them.

The attitudes that parents and staff hold are also likely to affect the ease with which they can work together. There are many different definitions of 'attitude', however, Schiffman and Kanuk (1996) describe an attitude as: a learned predisposition to behave in a consistently favourable or unfavourable way with respect to a given object. Atitudes may be described as 'implicit' (unconscious but having effects on behaviour) and 'explicit' (those which individuals recognise and acknowledge). The formation and development of attitudes is a continuous process, as knowledge and experience interact with existing attitudes and can change, modify or deepen these (Schiffman and Kanuk 1996). The attitudes that staff and families hold in relation to a vast range of things will affect their working relationship. However, what is perhaps the most important aspect of staff's attitudes for parents is the attitude they have towards them and their child, as people and as a family (Hewitt-Taylor 2007). This is closely related to their acceptance of and respect for the family's value system, and the values which individuals in the family hold.

Regardless of whether staff hold the same beliefs, values and opinions as families, being nonjudgemental of the family and valuing them as individuals and as a family unit is an attitude that is likely to facilitate the most effective working relationship. This includes staff developing respect for the values which the family hold, even where these are not their own. This development of a relationship in which respect exists, and where support is provided that genuinely aims to be in line with the child and family's values is essential in reducing the intrusion which staff create in the family's home and life.

RESPECT

The development of respect between staff and families is essential if high-quality support is to be provided. Mok (2005:274) defines respect as 'giving a person appropriate weight to the fact that he or she is a person and being willing to constrain ones behaviour in a manner required by that fact.' Respecting someone as a person means regarding them as possessing basic human dignity. This creates certain moral constraints on the actions which should be taken towards individuals and claims on how they should be treated. Respect for families applies not only to the person, but also to their surroundings, personal belongings, and others around them. This will be discussed in more detail in Chapter 5, in relation to working in the family home. However, respecting children, young people and their families, and treating them with the dignity and consideration they deserve as people is a mainstay of developing good working relationships and providing support that is beneficial to them.

The need for staff to be respectful of children, young people, and their families is undisputed, and forms a part of the professional obligation of a Registered Nurse (Nursing and Midwifery Council 2004). However, to facilitate optimum working, this respect needs to be mutual. Children, young people and their families should also show respect for the staff who work with them. The rights of staff are discussed in more detail in Chapter 8, but the principle of mutual respect means that families should afford staff consideration and dignity as human beings, and take into account the constraints that their values, beliefs and priorities and requirements of employment place on them. This may require open dialogue, and explicit decisions regarding how expectations and values can be managed and the reasons why staff may be unable to be involved in some activities or practices. The distinction between staff rejecting or questioning children, young people, and their parents' decision making, and staff being constrained by the requirements of their employer or their own values and beliefs should be made clear (Hewitt-Taylor 2007).

Case study

Parveen is 12. She cannot move independently, requires assistance in all her daily activities, has a tracheostomy and requires assisted ventilation.

Parveen enjoys spending time with her peers, and dislikes having a carer present when she is with them. When her family care for her, they often leave her with her friends, who can call them from a nearby location (such as the room next to the one she is in) if needed. However, the agreement which the Primary Care Trust have is that their staff will be with Parveen, providing constant supervision for her because she requires assisted ventilation. The staff who are employed by the Primary Care Trust are therefore not happy to leave her with her friends as the family do. Parveen finds it intrusive, but the staff who are employed to support her are uncomfortable over their position should her tracheostomy block, her ventilator become disconnected, or she need assistance when they are not there and her friends, who are around Parveen's age, fail to alert them. These concerns have led to discussions between the family and the nursing team regarding the position of each party, and an agreement has been drawn up regarding Parveen being left alone with friends, so that the expectations and responsibilities of all parties are clear. Staff are now able to leave her with her friends in certain circumstances, without fear of the consequences.

RESPECT FOR PARENTS' RESPONSIBILITY FOR THEIR CHILD

One aspect of the relationship between parents and staff which may be more challenging when working closely in the family home than in other circumstances is respecting parents' right to decision making about their child. The length of time over which support is likely to be provided, and the situations in which staff are likely to be involved will be more direct and continuous than on brief visits to the family home (Farasat and Hewitt-Taylor 2007). This may include the way in which children are expected to behave, and child discipline.

Although their remit is to provide support for families in caring for their child, in most cases staff are not employed for the purpose of providing unsolicited advice on general childcare issues. This can be a very sensitive area and staff should be aware that parents' childcare practices may be subject to comments and advice which are unrelated to their child's medical or technical needs, and which would not be made if they did not require assistance with their child's health needs. Unless this is within the specific remit of staff, or parents seek advice from them, staff giving unsolicited advice or opinions on childcare practices is not normally helpful and may be seen by parents as intrusive, and insulting. Whilst staff report that this can be uncomfortable at times, there is a need to recognise that all parents have different practices, and unless these constitute harm to the child, are not the place of other people to alter (Farasat and Hewitt-Taylor 2007).

Although staff should not offer unsolicited advice on general childcare issues, this may be difficult in practice, especially when working closely with families whose child rearing beliefs and practices are greatly at odds with one's own. Where practices are not something that staff can condone, or which they do not feel able to be involved in, a part of mutual respect and nonjudgemental behaviour includes this being discussed. Whilst staff should not be judgemental of parents, neither are they obliged to participate in situations and practices with which they feel uncomfortable or which they consider to be outside their remit. There may be times when facilitation is necessary to enable staff and parents to work together, and agreeing the way in which staff can support the child and family without compromising themselves.

Whilst the mainstay of working with parents is respecting their expertise in their child, their values and priorities, it is also important to be aware of the responsibilities held by each party. For parents, having parental responsibility for a child means assuming all the rights, duties, powers, responsibilities and authority that a parent of a child has by law (Department of Health 2004b). Those who have parental responsibility have the right to bring the child up according to their values, priorities and beliefs, and culture. However, there may be situations where this is harmful to the child, and professionals have a duty of care to every child with whom they work. The child's safety and best interests usually override all other considerations. This is discussed in more detail in Chapter 8, but is an area where lack of clarity may exist, and where the limits of acceptable parenting may give concern to some practitioners. The assertion that parents' rights should be respected is not a reason to neglect protecting children or vulnerable individuals. There should be very clear mechanisms and processes through which staff can seek support and discuss any childcare practices that cause them concern.

TRUST

The development of a relationship in which there is respect and openness is the most likely to create a relationship of trust. The existence of trust, like respect, does not imply that families and staff agree on everything, Rather, it means that the family's wishes, values, beliefs and priorities are known and respected by staff, that any limits to what staff are able to do or participate in is known to families and that both parties are aware that concerns or differences of opinion will be dealt with openly.

The mainstay of a good working relationship is therefore that there is respect and trust between staff and families. This is not easy to develop, and in order for it to be achieved, it is usually necessary for families and staff to have time to develop a relationship and system of working together. Unsurprisingly, the opportunity for staff to work consistently with children and their families has been identified as important in developing an optimum working relationship (Kirk 2001) and systems for providing support should aim to allow this. However, as Chapter 10 identifies, the problems inherent in recruiting and retaining staff may make this very difficult to achieve (Hewitt-Taylor 2007). In addition, consistent support by someone with whom the family do not get on well is unlikely to be helpful. Again, this is something that the provision of support should seek to address but which may be problematic where staff recruitment and retention is difficult, or where staff have to provide care across a number of families, all of whom they may not get on well with (Hewitt-Taylor 2007). Despite the difficulties in achieving these goals, they merit considerable attention in service planning because of the impact they have on the quality of the support provided.

Case study

Christine and Susan usually hold Tom whilst he goes to sleep, sing to him, and put him into his cot once he has settled. On one occasion, when Tom was having difficulty settling for the night, the carer on duty advised Christine to: 'Just put him down, and leave him for five minutes, to see if he will settle. You shouldn't hold him all the time, you're just making a rod for your own back.' This is not in line with how the couple see their relationship with their child, and how they want to care for him. Christine explained:

'I didn't ask for staff to come and advise me on how to bring Tom up. How to care for him. We just need them to be with him at night so we can get some sleep. She has no right to tell me what to do with my child, unless I ask her, which I didn't. That is my decision. She hasn't sat by his bed while he has been critically ill, willing him to live. She hasn't any idea what we have been through with Tom, and what we feel for him. So, to say when I should or should not cuddle him is completely inappropriate. Since she said that, when she is with Tom, we can't sleep. We know that if he is unsettled, or unhappy, she won't pick him up and cuddle him, and comfort him, like we would. She is very good, technically. If the ventilator alarms when she is there, I wouldn't worry, because she knows what to do, and she does it, but I don't trust her to care for him like I do most of the others. Now, when she looks after him, we don't sleep, because we worry, is he unhappy, is he unsettled, and is she is just ignoring him because she thinks that's what should be done.'

BOUNDARIES IN PROFESSIONAL RELATIONSHIPS

A part of staff and families establishing an effective working relationship is developing appropriate personal and professional boundaries (Samwell 2005). Boundaries are described by the Nursing and Midwifery Council (2002:5) as 'the limits of behaviour which allow a client and a registrant to engage safely in a therapeutic caring relationship'.

Although the relationship that staff develop with clients is often the most important or satisfying part of nursing work, it is also an area in which difficulties can arise. Working with children and families in their homes often brings staff into closer contact with them, and does not create the same inhibition on involvement with them that working in a hospital environment does. Whilst it necessitates the development of a good working relationship, it also creates a greater potential for personal bonds to be formed and for nurses to identify closely with families and their situation (Samwell 2005). This can be a positive step in enabling staff to provide support which sees the child, young person and their family as people and respecting them and their priorities and values. However, it can also become problematic in terms of the boundaries required for effective working and staff have described becoming too close to families in a way which is not helpful to either party (Hewitt-Taylor 2007).

The Nursing and Midwifery Council (2002) describe the intended relationship between registrants and their clients as being a therapeutic caring relationship focused on meeting the health or care needs of the client. This does not imply that nurses who work with children and young people who have complex health needs should not see beyond the child or young person's healthcare needs, or seek to provide support that facilitates their needs as a person and as a part of their family. What it does mean is that staff must always keep in mind that their purpose is to provide the care or support which the child or young person and family needs, wants, or sees as a priority. Whilst the support which is provided should aim to embrace all their needs, staff should not impose themselves, in any way, on the child, young person or their family or use their position in any other way than to provide the care or support which the child, young person, or family has requested. Whilst this may seem relatively clear-cut, there are many grey areas related to involvement with children, young people and their families, and, particularly when staff are working closely with a family, in their home, it may be easy to overstep therapeutic boundaries.

The type of work that staff are engaged in, and the time they spend with families means that it can be very difficult to achieve the right balance of involvement, and for each party to give the right signals about the level of involvement they want and the roles they see themselves as playing. Samwell (2005) describes how easy it is for staff who work closely with families in their homes to inadvertently give the wrong impression about their intended or desired level of involvement, for example by giving too much information about their personal lives in casual conversation. It is also relatively easy for misunderstandings to occur regarding what each party sees as the relationship. For example, parents may perceive that staff have become their friends: because they seem to get on well, because of the information they each disclose about themselves, because of the time they spend together, or their apparent shared concern about the child. In contrast, staff may not see parents as their friends, but rather consider their involvement to be a part of their job, related solely to their work persona (Samwell 2005). Equally, staff may make the same error of judgement over whether families see them as friends. As Samwell (2005) identifies, the skills involved in communicating an interest in and commitment to families, being attentive to the needs of the child or young person and their family as people, and establishing trust without overstepping professional boundaries is possibly the most difficult part of working closely with families.

If very close bonds do form between staff and families, when staff move on from their job the bond may be broken or modified, which can be hurtful for the family, and for staff where they have themselves become dependent on the family (Samwell 2005). This is especially likely where one party has seen their relationship differently from the other. Where staff become too involved in a family's life, this may be problematic for them because their private time and emotional energy becomes absorbed by a commitment to the family to the exclusion of other aspects of their life (Samwell 2005). Equally, where staff want to become more involved than the family find helpful (often with good intentions of providing high-quality, person-centred support which shows an interest in the family), families may find this intrusive and claustrophobic (Hewitt-Taylor 2007).

The level of everyday involvement that staff inevitably have with a family with whom they work closely, and the workload which many families have to juggle, may make nurses want to solve their problems for them. However, it is important to avoid establishing a relationship that encourages families to be dependent on individual staff, and their views, opinions, or solutions to problems (Samwell 2005). This may be very difficult for staff, because most people who enter 'caring' professions want to assist others. However, as is discussed in other chapters, what is best for one person or family will not be best for another, and the role that staff should usually take on is therefore to assist families to identify what their wishes and preferences are, and to find ways in which these might be achieved or met. The intention should be to enable children, young people and their families to develop autonomy, not dependence on individual staff. Despite the temptation to solve problems for children, young people and their families, this is not likely to be helpful for them in the long term. There also can be a problem for families where staff have a 'need to be needed' as well as a desire to assist families (Samwell 2005). This can result in staff imposing their services in a way that families find domineering, unhelpful and intrusive and which may be disempowering or harmful to them.

Managing this balance of involvement and caring with over-involvement and intrusion requires self-awareness by staff, and insight into whose needs are being met when they become involved with a family (Samwell 2005). The Nursing and Midwifery Council (2002:5) state that 'Moving the focus of care away from meeting clients' needs towards meeting the registrant's own needs is an unacceptable abuse of power.' Thus, engaging a relationship in which a staff members' need to be needed or to help the family is greater than their desire to meet the child or young person and their family's needs as identified by them could be seen as a departure from acceptable professional conduct.

Case study

Parveen has carers to support her every night, whilst she is at school, and short-break care 24 hours a day one weekend in six. Her family do not want to develop a close relationship with her carers. They prefer the time they have from carers to be clearly focused on enabling Parveen to be safe, cared for, and for the weekends when they have short-break care to enable her to develop relationships and interests with her peers, as other girls of her age would. However, Parveen's mother explains: 'We have one carer who always wants to chat about what we have done that day, and what she has done that day. I find that irritating really. I don't really want the carers to be a part of our life as a family. I do want them to tell me about what Parveen has done at school, anything we need to know about her, because they are there for her. But I am not here to listen to what she (the carer) did at home, what is happening in her life. I am getting to dread her arriving. She spends at least 40 minutes just chatting, about herself mostly, and her opinions. I just want to get on with everything I have to do. I waste the first 40 minutes of time which I am given supposedly to help me, and to mean I can get to bed, listening to her problems, hearing about her life. So, although she is meant to be here for nine hours, we only get seven. She is meant to start work at 10 for a night shift. I want to go to bed, because I have to be up again at six to help get Parveen ready for school, not chat to her.'

Although staff being over-involved with families may be a problem, there are also likely to be situations in which a member of staff and family do not get on well enough to develop a good working relationship. The personalities of staff and families may be incompatible, or their beliefs or values incongruent and unreconcilable. This is possible in all healthcare settings and encounters. However, it is perhaps a more important consideration when the care or support provided will be for many hours, every day, long term, in the family home, and where staff cannot be as easily directed to care for another family as they can in ward settings.

Staff working in the family home and families who require support at home have the same right to be treated without prejudice as staff and families in any other setting, as will be discussed in more depth in Chapter 8. However, there may be situations where it is in the best interests of all parties that staff do not work with a particular family, because they cannot work well together and a continuation of involvement is in nobody's best interests. Something which staff, families and service providers need to recognise is that a large part of working in the home is being able to form a balanced relationship with the family. If this cannot be achieved, and is to the detriment of the provision of support, the situation is not therapeutic. Furthermore, this should not be seen as insulting to either party, rather an acknowledgement of the uniqueness of human beings and the complexity of working closely with other people, in what is effectively a very intimate setting.

WORKING WITH PARENTS WHO ARE EXPERTS

Parents whose children have complex and continuing health needs are usually experts in their child's medical, technical and healthcare requirements. They uniquely know about their child's condition, how they respond to a range of situations, how they respond to various therapeutic interventions, and, perhaps most vitally, know their child as a person (Kirk et al. 2005; Hewitt-Taylor 2007). They are experts in every aspect of their child and their care and in how their child's complex health needs can be managed in the context of the family as a whole.

Parents whose children have complex and continuing health needs, and children and young people themselves, are often far more knowledgeable about the disease processes associated with their condition, the treatment which they need, the practicalities and intricacies of their care and management than many healthcare professionals. Parents in this situation regularly perform procedures for their children that are outside the knowledge or experience of some healthcare staff and are often involved in teaching professionals about these (Glendinning and Kirk 2000; Department of Health 2001b). They also become experts in monitoring their child's condition and are usually able to detect changes in their state of health and well-being earlier than professionals, using intuition and in-depth knowledge of their child rather than measurable parameters or concrete clinical signs as their guides (Judson 2004; Kirk et al. 2005). This is combined with what some parents describe as a 'sixth sense' for communicating with their child, but which also enables them to know when something unmeasurable, and often hardly definable, but definite, is wrong (Hewitt-Taylor 2007).

The expertise that anyone who has a long-term condition has in their own condition and needs is recognised in healthcare policy. The Department of Health (2001b) describes how patients generally have expertise in their personal experience of health and illness, social circumstances, attitudes to risk, values and preferences, whilst healthcare professionals have expertise in diagnosis, disease processes, prognosis, treatment options and outcome probabilities. Whilst children or young people who have complex health needs and their parents have this expertise in their own experiences, values and priorities, they are often also well informed about the disease processes, treatment options and practicalities of healthcare associated with their condition. The widespread availability of a plethora of electronic medical resources adds to their ability to gain information that might traditionally have been seen as the province of healthcare staff (Hewitt-Taylor 2006). This means that the expectations regarding the division of 'expertise' may be less clear-cut than is often suggested, and may make discussions more threatening for professionals, as it means that children, young people and their families are more likely to be able to challenge and debate their knowledge and views (Glendinning and Kirk 2000).

Although professionals may find this change in established roles threatening, parents do not generally object to professionals having limited knowledge about their child's condition (provided this is outside their usual remit). Rather, they value professionals who admit the limitations in their knowledge, and the knowledge of medicine as a whole. This honesty, provided it is perceived as open sharing of information rather than unconcern or indifference, can form the basis for a trusting relationship. In this way, each party contributes their knowledge, experience and views, and open and honest discussion can occur with the intention of ascertaining what is best for the child or young person (Kirk and Glendinning 2004; Hewitt-Taylor 2007). However, some parents feel that professionals find their knowledge threatening. In addition, their expertise is not always fully acknowledged and their views sometimes ignored or dismissed. This is particularly so where their experiential and intuitive knowledge contrasts with the objective, scientific knowledge with which healthcare professionals are more familiar and to which they appear to attach greater value (Kirk and Glendinning 2004; Kirk et al. 2005). In contrast, children, young people and their families are expected to value the objective, scientific knowledge contributed by professionals.

Case study

Susan and Christine can tell when Tom is beginning to feel uncomfortable, and can usually identify the cause, for example, if he is not in a comfortable position, if he needs suction, or if his feed is causing him discomfort. Although he cannot make very clear vocal sounds, they can tell by his facial expressions and body posture what he wants to communicate. Susan explains that: 'I can tell, I just know, how he is feeling, whether he's tired, or uncomfortable, or bored. I can tell the difference in his expression, how he holds me, or how he lies against me, how he responds. Often it's just the way he looks at me. Sometimes there's just something in his eyes that means he isn't quite right. Last time he got sick, I knew three days before anyone believed me. There was nothing visible, nothing I could get anyone to listen to, but I knew. He was just not comfortable. He couldn't get comfortable, and was coughing a bit more than usual, but more than anything it was just something I felt from how he was. By the time he had a fever, and had masses of secretions, and was obviously ill, it was too late, he ended up in PICU. If they'd listened to us, when we said something wasn't right, well, maybe it wouldn't have made a difference, because they didn't have much to go on to treat, but because we couldn't say exactly, in medical terms, what was wrong, it was as if we were just panicking, making a fuss, being worriers.'

Although parents are generally the experts in their child's condition, management and care, and this should be respected, this does not absolve healthcare professionals of responsibility for their own knowledge and for contributing this to the child or young person's care. Some parents have identified that whilst they are the experts in their own child's care needs, they are not medically trained and look to professionals to respond appropriately when they reach the limits of their knowledge. This includes when new situations arise or when new procedures or care are needed (Hewitt-Taylor 2007). The skill of working with expert parents requires a combination of listening to, believing and acting on parental expertise, concerns or observations, and combining this with the knowledge and expertise that professionals have, in order to reach a solution. Whilst parents become experts in their child's care, this takes time to develop and professionals have an important role in working in partnership and supporting them, to facilitate the development of expertise, and to contribute from their own knowledge base as well as learning from parents.

A challenge for professionals is, therefore, to work in partnership with children, young people and their families, sharing and valuing the knowledge, skills, and resources which all parties contribute. Donaldson (2003) suggests that achieving this type of partnership working is not easy, and that it requires changes in the attitudes and modes of interaction of many healthcare professionals and service users. It needs consistent negotiation, effort, honesty and respect on all sides, with open communication and flexibility over what each party may see as their role.

ENABLING AND SUPPORTING PARENTS TO ACCESS AND ACCEPT SUPPORT

Although parents are generally the experts in their child's care, the practicalities of this can be exhausting and isolating. Whilst the day-to-day practical support that staff provide may ease parents' physical burden, other services, facilities and resources may also be useful for them. This may include facilities and services within Health Services, Social Services, and from external agencies, for example, charitable organisations, support groups and specialist organisations. One aspect of offering support to families may be providing children, young people and their families with information on the available resources, and enabling them to access these types of support if they wish to do so.

Support organisations may be very helpful for families in terms of lessening the isolation and stigmatisation they may feel, and in creating a sense of belonging. Where so many elements of society appear to devalue their children, parents may find that support organisations are a place where they can feel safe and where they and their child are understood and valued. They may also be a useful place for parents to share ideas and strategies, and where they can give, as well as receive support and assistance (Davies and Hall 2005). Staff may be able to recommend organisations that have the potential to be helpful for families in this respect. Examples of such organisations and how to access them can be seen in Appendix 1.

There is also evidence that many parents are unaware of or fail to claim the state benefits to which they are entitled or to apply for funds which might be available to them (Department of Health 2004a; Hewitt-Taylor 2007). Nursing staff may not be aware of all the benefits or allowances to which parents may be entitled, or their rights at work, (such as their right to flexible working) (Contact a Family 2004a). However, they may be able to refer parents to agencies who can provide them with information, or to advise parents on organisations or individuals who may be of assistance in this respect.

As well as recommending and referring families to services or facilities, staff should be aware of the reasons why individuals and families may not seek or be reluctant to accept support. Some families may prefer to manage alone, and may consider that the intrusion that accessing support would necessitate would be more problematic than the workload of caring for their child. This should be respected, but channels left open for them to seek support in the future (Brett 2004). In other situations, families may desire some assistance, but appear reluctant to seek or accept this. Understanding some of the reasons for this may enable staff to assist families to access or accept support which might be beneficial to them.

Brett (2004) describes how the pervading attitudes of society which place having a disabled child as a negative experience may mean that parents are disinclined to access support. For some families, this builds on the implication that their child is a burden with which they require assistance, rather than a child whom they love and value. A part of showing the value they attach to their child is caring for them. They may also fear that staff who assist with their child may, like society as a whole, not value them. Asking for support can be seen by some parents as an admission of failure, or letting their child down, especially given society's expectations of parents and attitudes towards disabled children. Seeking support can also represent a form of loss for parents, including loss of complete autonomy, loss of sole responsibility for their child and loss of their role (Brett 2004). Acknowledging the complexity of factors that influence parents' decisions over whether or not to seek support and the type of support which they prefer is valuable in assisting them to access the level of support which is right for them at any given time (Brett 2004).

UNDERSTANDING AND WORKING WITH THE FAMILY'S EXPECTATIONS

Parents and professionals may have different expectations of a child or young person, different views about their likely outcomes, different perceptions of what outcomes are important, and the level and type of interventions which are appropriate or helpful. In some situations, staff may consider that parents have unrealistic expectations for or of their child. In other situations, staff may see parents as apparently unaccountably lacking in optimism, for example in relation to new or innovative therapies (Farnalls and Rennick 2003).

Developing a good working relationship with families and discussing their perceptions and priorities with them may enable staff to gain a better understanding of why they hold certain views or appear to respond in given ways to their situation. This may also create the opportunity for staff to challenge their own thinking and perceptions of what is important. For example, Farnalls and Rennick (2003) found that when a new therapy was offered to parents whose children suffered from severe epilepsy, many seemed cautious in their hopes, whereas professionals were generally enthusiastic about its potential benefits. However, it became clear that after years of disappointed hopes, instead of placing high hopes on this new possibility many parents made a conscious effort to control their expectations, to protect themselves against disappointment. Equally, parents may reframe time and redefine their priorities and expectations in order to manage their child's needs. This may mean that staff see them as having unrealistic expectations when in fact they simply have different goals, ways of viewing the world, and views on what matters for their child, and their quality of life. Their knowledge of their child as a person and the value of the relationship which they have with them, based on the present, not the future, often enables parents to have a different view of the value and quality of many aspects of their life than staff, however closely they work with the child. They may value the present point in time, because the future is largely unknown.

Case study

Christine describes how: 'I know people at work, and our families and staff at the hospital wonder, why do we bother? Not why do we bother to care for Tom, but why, when he gets sick, why are we so upset if people are slow to pick up on things. Why are we so obsessed with him, I suppose. I heard one nurse saying last time he was in: 'Well, long term, he's not going anywhere, is he?' We are realistic. We know he isn't going to live as long as other children. It's been a hard process, but we do know he is not going to even outlive us. We are not naïve. We do know. But we also know that right now, he is here with us, and he enjoys his life and we love him, and his company. He enjoys so many things. He enjoys his bath, he loves being splashed. He loves being tickled. He absolutely adores us making silly faces at him. He nearly chokes his trache tube out if we both pull faces at him at once. He is so happy when we go to the park and feed the ducks, and watch the kites flying and he loves seeing other children on the swings. He has so many pleasures and we have so much pleasure with him. So, if we were talking about major surgery, and he would be in pain, and maybe not have the quality of life he has now, then that might be different. But to just not treat a chest infection, or be so slow in picking up on it, when he still enjoys so many things and when we enjoy being with him and seeing him enjoy himself so much. To us, that is wrong. We don't know how long he will be with us, so we enjoy every day. We don't plan 'Well, what will he do when he's 20?' because we know he won't be 20. So we don't see the point in other people doing that either, or making that a reason to decide on whether he should be allowed to enjoy now. And yes, we are obsessed by him, because we don't think we will be together for very long. Going back to the night nurse who wanted us to not cuddle him. We don't know how many cuddles we've got. Every one is precious.'

SUMMARY

Working closely, on a regular basis, with children and young people who have complex and continuing health needs and their parents can be very rewarding but can also present staff and families with very specific challenges. Negotiating the role that staff will take in the child or young person's care and support, the house rules and the relationship which they will have with the family with whom they work is very different and more intense than the negotiation needed in most other settings.

Developing effective working relationships with children, young people and their parents requires staff to respect them as people, their values, priorities, and home. It also requires them to respect parents' childcare practices and their responsibility for their child, to be able to learn from parents, and engage in a relationship of mutual sharing of knowledge, skills, and experience, for the benefit of the child. The relationship should aim to facilitate what the child, young person and their family want and to enable them to function as a family with as little as possible intrusion whilst also supporting them.

The stereotypical view of families of disabled children being 'in need' is not helpful, as it implies that any assistance offered to them will be beneficial (Barr and Millar 2003). What is more appropriate is to recognise that whilst parents may need assistance with their child's care, this support is only required because of the extraordinary workload they have and should be aimed at enabling them and their family to enjoy their relationship with their child, in the way that they want to.

Chapter 5
Working in the Family Home

There is a general belief that children and young people benefit from being in the home environment (Department of Health 2004a). However, when children or young people have complex health needs this often places a significant workload on their families, particularly their parents (Hewitt-Taylor 2007). Although families generally want to do everything possible to enable their child to live at home, it may be impossible for them to achieve this without some support from health and social care professionals. The amount and type of support families need or want varies, as will be discussed in Chapter 10, but may involve staff spending many hours in the family home. Parents may require support for a few hours on an irregular basis, regular overnight support so that they can sleep, or as much as 24-hour a day assistance.

Whatever the amount and type of support that families receive, having a visitor in their home often constitutes an intrusion to their life and creates a number of specific issues which staff must consider and manage. This chapter discusses some of these issues.

BEING A VISITOR IN ONE'S OWN WORKPLACE

A major consideration for staff who support children and young people in their home is that they are working in the family's living place, and in their lives (Farasat and Hewitt-Taylor 2007). Unlike staff who carry out a series of short visits to a variety of homes, with a base to which they return in between, for many staff who provide the day-to-day support for children who have complex health needs and their families, their permanent workplace is someone else's house and home. This creates specific issues and considerations, which other staff do not have. It entails them recognising the need to be 'good guests' as all staff involved in community healthcare must. However, the length and frequency of their stay means that the potential for them to outstay or overstep their welcome and intrude on the family's life is greater than for those visiting for short periods of time or on an occasional basis (Farasat and Hewitt-Taylor 2007).

Chapter 4 discussed the need for staff to respect families, and this applies equally to respecting their home and how they live, and not imposing their own values, beliefs or opinions on them or on their living space. It is important for staff to be respectful of and responsive to the various meanings which individuals attach to the concept of 'home' and to accept what, for each family, is a safe and individual place (Kelly and Uddin 2005). In the same way that Chapter 4 described the need to avoid intruding on the family, their home should not be intruded upon.

INTRUSION VERSUS SUPPORT

Despite being capable of and willing to care for their child, many parents require assistance to manage the practical demands of their care as well as the other essential aspects of their lives: housework, shopping, caring for other siblings, and getting enough sleep to provide care for their child during the day. The provision of staff to assist families in their child's care on a day-to-day basis is therefore often essential to enable children and young people who have complex and continuing health needs to live at home. However, the presence of staff in their home has a great potential to intrude on families. They have a person who was often previously unknown to them, and not selected by them, visiting their home, regularly, and often for many hours (Valkenier et al. 2002). Families are effectively obliged to share their lives and houses with a stranger, and in some cases, to have a stranger in their lives 24 hours a day.

Although staff and families may take various measures to minimise the intrusion which staff, almost of necessity, create, many houses are not sufficiently spacious to easily accommodate an additional adult or adults. Perhaps the most important part of minimising intrusion is staff recognising that for many families they will always be unwelcome, not personally, and not with ingratitude, but because most families would prefer not to require assistance, and the necessary intrusion which this creates (Hewitt-Taylor 2007).

The concept of privacy has been alluded to in Chapter 1 in relation to children's rights, and the privacy for the whole family can be an issue when staff are regularly in their home (Magnusson et al. 2002). Families are required to expose their lifestyle, relationships, and what for them constitutes 'home' to others. Families may feel the need to maintain a level of tidiness and cleanliness in their homes which is stressful and not expected of other families, because of having constant visitors, not because this creates an environment which they enjoy living in (Hewitt-Taylor 2007). Some families may feel that every aspect of their home and life is under scrutiny and that observations, comments or questions about their home are intrusive, even if made in the spirit of casual conversation. For other families, such conversations may convey an interest in and engagement with them that they appreciate. One of the challenges for staff who work in families' homes is to work with families whose preferences about their relationship with staff and the way in which they want them to be involved in their home and life will be highly individual (Hewitt-Taylor 2007).

Case study

Aki is nine. He needs assisted ventilation at night. His parents, Chieri and Makito have carers to look after him every night, because he needs someone to make sure that his ventilator is working correctly, and to attend to any alarms. Chieri explains: 'Really, I am not very happy to have someone else in my house every night, but we can't stay up all night and then all day as well. I don't like someone else being here, forming opinions, even if they don't say anything. The other day one of the carers said to me: "I like working here. Your house is so nice and peaceful." It was compliment, but it made me think, I wonder what else they notice, and think, and talk about amongst themselves.

'They are mostly nice people, and their coming means that I can get some sleep, but it does also create work for me. I have to clean the house every day, especially Aki's room, because I don't want them to get a bad impression of my house and they need to work in a nice environment. I have to have everything looking nice. I have to make sure we have washed up before they arrive. Aki goes to bed at about 8.30 and I need to have everything done by then because I sit with him until they arrive. I have to make sure there is coffee, tea, sugar and milk for them. If it wasn't for having to sleep, it would almost be more work than it's worth.'

By being in a family's home, staff are privy to intimate knowledge about them, their relationships, their way of life and stressors (Dimond 2000). When a third party is present in the home, family relationships have to be conducted in an environment that is not private and they may feel unable to exchange views, argue and enjoy intimacy as other families do. It may be difficult to have privacy for conversations and telephone calls (for business, financial and personal or family matters) and these may therefore be more constrained. The entire life of a family who have a member of staff in their home for significant periods of the day is open to observation by other people. These are often individuals with whom they have not yet had the chance to develop a relationship, or trust. Some parents describe this as like 'living in a goldfish bowl' (Hewitt- Taylor 2007).

Where support is required at night, parents may even feel a lack of privacy when they sleep, and in their bedrooms, particularly if staff may have to seek advice from them during the night. Some parents describe measures which may be useful in overcoming this, such as installing call bells or intercoms so that staff do not need to visit their rooms (Hewitt-Taylor 2007). Even so, depending on the design of the house, and how well individuals sleep, some people find that the slightest action by staff at night, and even the awareness that someone else is awake in their house, disrupts their sleep (Hewitt-Taylor 2007).

Having a third party in the home may mean that families do not feel relaxed and at ease in their own home, and lack personal space (Hewitt-Taylor 2007). As well as their physical privacy being interrupted, the child or young person and their family may find that their emotional privacy is limited. They may have nowhere completely private to explore or give vent to their own emotions, and may feel uncomfortable or threatened if staff see them expressing their feelings (Brett 2004). Whilst staff may be a source of emotional support, if individuals prefer to work through their feelings alone, having a member of staff constantly in their home may be problematic. For staff, a great challenge can be knowing when to offer emotional support, and when this actually constitutes unwelcome intrusion on a person's privacy which another parent would not be subject to.

Whilst on one hand the provision of support may give parents the opportunity to go out, it may also decrease their social opportunities because visits from family and friends have to either take place in the presence of a third party, or the family plan for visitors to come at times when a carer is not present. As discussed in Chapter 3, this can make it more difficult for parents whose child has complex health needs to stay in contact with friends and relations than it is for other parents, and although they have support in caring for their child, they may lose friendships and other forms of support which are important to them.

Case study

Jake, who is now two, was born prematurely, and has some residual lung damage which means he requires CPAP all the time. He also has a gastrostomy, via which he receives overnight feeds, and has frequent seizures. His parents, Hannah and Charles have two other children: Lauren aged 3½ and Sarah aged 5. They live in a three bedroom terraced house, with a lounge/dining room, a small kitchen, and a small garden. Charles works shifts, including night shifts. Hannah used to work part time, but left work after Jake was born. The family have 24-hour support to assist them with Jake's care.

As the family only have one downstairs room, there is nowhere except the bedrooms which are not Jake's and where his parents can go for privacy. When Charles is on night duty, Hannah has nowhere in the house where she can go to be alone, or to have privacy except for Lauren and Sarah's room. Even when she can use their bedroom sound travels very easily in the house and Hannah feels that staff can hear every phone call, see anyone who calls to the house and hear what they say. She explains: 'Although it looks as if we have a big house, it isn't that much room, for three adults and three children, one of whom is on CPAP. It does feel crowded. Even though the staff are very tactful, you never feel you can guarantee someone won't overhear you or walk in on you.' Charles finds it difficult to sleep in the day, because he can hear the care staff.

Charles and Hannah generally get on well with the care staff, but sometimes find it very claustrophobic. Hannah describes how: 'We do appreciate the help, because we get a lot really, and it means Jake can be with us, but I feel like I always have to be on my best behaviour, I always have to be friendly and chatty. I feel as if I have no life just as me. I am never going to be just me, I always have someone here, who I have to be on my best behaviour for. When my friend called round the other day, I felt I had to introduce her to the carer, and then they had a chat, and then she kept joining in our conversation, and it was like, I can't even just have my friends round and talk to them.'

For some people, having a member of staff in the house means that information about a health need has to be disclosed, which might not otherwise be necessary, because the presence of care staff has to be accounted for (Hewitt-Taylor 2007). For instance, a member of staff visiting the home may mean that visitors or neighbours become aware that someone in the family has a health problem. Whilst this is inevitable, it means that the family's private life is not as secure as it might otherwise be and even a member of staff's car parked in the road can be an intrusion into their lives and give information to their neighbours which they would prefer to keep private.

When they care for their child at home, parents do not need to 'parent in public' in the way that they would in hospital. However, when healthcare staff are frequently in the family home and assisting in their child's day-to-day care, their childcare practices become open to observation by outsiders. Parents, particularly new parents, may have to develop their relationship with their child, their childcare skills, and work out how to manage caring for their child at home in the presence of others. Whilst the support which they are given may be valuable, it can also mean that parents feel observed, and ill at ease, and do not have the privacy which other parents have to develop their unique relationship with their child, and to develop the style of parenting and lifestyle which best suits them and their child (Hewitt-Taylor 2007).

As discussed in Chapter 3, becoming a parent can be a stressful as well as exciting time. Having to undergo this learning curve, and the additional learning involved in having a child who has complex health needs in the presence of relative strangers, (particularly strangers who may be perceived as childcare workers, professionals or experts), can be difficult, albeit unavoidable. Parents may fear criticism, especially from professionals, and may also be subjected to advice about basic childcare which, whilst well intentioned, may be contradictory, unhelpful and overwhelming.

Case study

Hannah has had a carer in the house permanently ever since Jake came home. She recalls: 'I never really felt that Jake was mine. I have always had a nurse here all night, and most of the day. I felt like I never really had time to just be me, with Jake and the girls, us all getting to know each other. First he was in hospital for ages, so we were rushing between here and there and getting to know him in the middle of a neonatal unit in front of staff, and just bringing the girls in for an hour or so. Then when he came home we had carers here. In one way I was lucky. I could bring Jake home, and I had someone to help me, because I couldn't have managed the other two and him alone. At the time the girls were three and 18 months, so I could never have juggled everything, but sometimes, I would just have liked to be alone with him. For us to be alone as a family, getting to know him too, without someone else there. If we asked, of course we could cancel the carers, but what I suppose I really miss is just being able to have time with the whole family, being just us, which I can't, because I can't juggle his needs and the girl's all on my own. Plus, you don't want to cancel care, because then they think you don't need it, and it might be reduced. And I do need it. It's just, I have never really felt Jake is mine the way I did with the girls.'

The siblings of a child whose needs mean that the family require support at home may also feel the intrusion of a third party in their lives and personal space. They may feel observed, that their relationship with their parents and brother or sister is open to scrutiny, and that visits from friends are affected by a member of care staff being present in their home. There have also been instances in which the way in which support is organised and implemented can make siblings feel unwanted and excluded in their own home. For example, if carers do not see working with siblings as being within their remit, or are not permitted to be alone with the child and their siblings, the child's brothers or sisters can be excluded from interactions with them and the family be effectively separated from them despite being in their own home (Hewitt-Taylor 2007). Those providing support should act in a way that includes siblings in their brother or sister's life, but also have to try to balance this inclusion with intrusion into siblings' lives.

Case study

Chieri now has two children, Aki and Emori. Emori is three years old, and he and Aki are very close. One morning Emori went into Aki's room early, to show him a new toy he wanted to play with. The carer asked Emori to leave the room, because she was only supposed to look after Aki, not have responsibility for other children. Aki had woken up by this time, and the carer discontinued his assisted ventilation. Aki said that he could look after his brother himself. However, by the this time Emori was very upset at having been told off, and because he wanted to be with his brother. Chieri explains: "I know they are not responsible for Emori, but he is three, he doesn't understand about employment rules. I think she could have just let him be, because Aki was waking up anyway, so she could have just helped him sort himself out, then Aki would have been able to play with Emori, and she (the carer) didn't even need to be there any more. Really, she didn't need to feel responsible for Emori. He wasn't interfering with Aki's ventilation. If any other three year old goes into his older brother's room, they just get on with it, they don't need an adult. Or she could have called me. But she sent him away. Told him he couldn't be with his brother."

STAFF SAFETY AND WELL-BEING IN THE WORKPLACE

Families who have staff working in their homes on a regular basis are likely to face situations and have to take into account factors, which other families do not. Likewise, the staff who work with them may also have concerns which they would not in other situations. As well as families having reduced privacy, working in the family home can reduce the privacy of staff. Staff have described feeling more 'on edge' in some homes than in others, and whilst families may feel observed, staff may also feel very closely observed by families, and uncomfortable in their work because of this (Hewitt-Taylor 2007). They may come to know the family in a way which is closer and more intimate than in other circumstances. This means that they are more likely than other staff to inadvertently disclose personal information to families which they later regret, or to become more involved with the family than they intended (Hewitt-Taylor 2007).

Whilst staff should respect families and their homes, this respect should be mutual, and staff should not have their safety and well-being compromised (Taylor and Donnelly 2006). The issues that staff may have to negotiate include use of facilities, where they can make drinks and meals, and the expected level of cleanliness in such areas. Discussions may include issues which those working in third-party premises or visiting homes for short periods of time do not have to negotiate, such as flushing toilets on night duty and balancing families' right to quiet with staff's need to carry out their work and, if necessary, communicate with other team members (Farasat and Hewitt-Taylor 2007; Hewitt-Taylor 2007). Whilst staff should respect the choices which families make regarding their home, and their environment, this can be problematic if the environment is not conducive to working or constitutes an unacceptable level of risk for staff.

The family have a right to maintain their home as they choose, but staff also have a right to safety at work. However, creating a safe working environment in the family home may not be straightforwad because, unless staff are employed directly by the family, their employer does not have control of the environment in the way that they do in, for example, a hospital. It may also be difficult to balance staff safety and respect for families' preferences and choices (Taylor and Donnelly 2006). Although this may apply to all community based work, where staff are in one house for a full shift on a regular basis, any issues in a particular home become more pronounced.

Health and safety regulations mean that employers have a duty of care to their employees, and this includes those who work in families' homes (Taylor and Donnelly 2006). There is a statutory duty (as set out in the Health and Safety at Work Act 1974) and a common law duty for employers to take reasonable care for the health and safety at work of their employees. These require the employer to ensure a safe premises, plant and equipment and a safe system of work (Dimond 1999). These regulations apply equally to private homes as any other work environment, and employers should have systems in place to ensure that the premises in which their staff work are safe. However, there are differences between what would be seen as a reasonable expectation of employers in the home and in a hospital environment. For example, there would be no liability for the employer for harm caused to the employee as a result of defective home maintenance unless the house were known to be in a dangerous condition that employees should not have been sent there. If staff are injured in such circumstances, they are usually dependent on the resources or insurance cover of the occupier or owner of the property, and should consider obtaining personal accident cover for working in other people's homes (Dimond 1999).

Requirements for safety in relation to moving and handling may present specific challenges when an individual is working in the family home. Many NHS Trusts have a 'no lifting' policy, and where staff care for a child or young person at home appropriate lifting and handling equipment (such as a hoist) is usually made available for the family and them. However, if an individual prefers manual lifting on the grounds of their perceived safety or dignity, the legal position that staff are in is not clear cut. Whilst health and safety regulations related to moving and handling usually protect staff, in care situations, it is expected that staff will take greater risks because of the human nature of their load (Griffith and Stevens 2004). Generally the health and safety of employees favours the use of mechanical methods of lifting, but there are circumstances where the balance would fall in favour of the individual's right to be lifted manually (Griffith and Stevens 2004). There is no absolute law on this issue, but staff should highlight to their employers any concerns they have, request appropriate training for their specific situation, and document any risks they are required to take and how they have sought to resolve these. To fulfill their duties, employers should develop manual handling policies and risk assessment strategies that strike a balance between risk and need in each individual case (Griffith and Stevens 2004).

Staff who work in the home may, as in any other workplace, encounter violence. However, when they are working in a family home, they are usually more isolated and cannot call on in-house security staff or their colleagues to assist them or raise the alarm. The employer's duty to their employees includes that of taking reasonable action to prevent them suffering harm as a result of violence towards them. Staff should be provided with appropriate training to assist them to deal with violence within the home and should not be expected to work in environments where they are known to be in danger. Staff also have a responsibility to ensure that colleagues and managers are notified about potential dangers and that any untoward incidents are documented (Dimond 1999). Staff may need to be provided with escorts to visit areas considered to be dangerous, and in exceptional cases, a home environment may not be safe for staff to work in because of violent family members, or violence against the family. Employees should make their employers aware of such risks, and employers have a responsibility to take all reasonable steps to ensure staff safety, including withdrawing staff from dangerous situations where this is the only option.

It may be useful for service providers and families to have service agreements in place to clarify the expectations of all parties and to formalise what has been deemed to be reasonable behaviour and a reasonable working environment by all concerned. This may include clarification over the family's rights, the rights of staff, and the consequences of certain decisions by families. For example, it may need to be made explicit that staff will leave the premises if asked to do so or if certain safety standards are not met, but that this will mean that responsibility for the care of the child rests with the family (Widdas et al. 2005).

Whilst families have a right to conduct their lives and relationships as they see fit and as best suits their preferences and values, the emotional atmosphere that their personalities and relationships create is a potential issue for staff who work in their homes. If families do not get on well, and there is an atmosphere of discontent or conflict in the home, this may be difficult for staff to work with. Staff may be called on to take sides in family arguments, and, whilst this is not a part of their role, they may be placed in difficult situations if this occurs on a regular basis. This may be an inevitable part of working in the family home, but is a consideration for home care staff which other staff may not face as regularly, or with such intensity.

Case study

Helen works with Eleanor, aged five, who requires assisted ventilation at night, and her mother, Carol. The staff are only reluctantly given access to facilities and describe the home environment as very unwelcoming and unfriendly. Carol lives alone with Eleanor, but has had a number of boyfriends over the past five years, many of whom staff have met and spoken to on arrival at the house. They are frequently verbally abusive towards Carol, and have very little to do with Eleanor. Occasionally when staff are present Carol or her boyfriend will try to include them in their arguments. It has been made clear to Carol that staff will not be drawn into such situations.

Carol's current boyfriend is often drunk when staff arrive, and is frequently insulting to them. Helen has expressed concerns about the work environment, and meetings have been held with Carol in which changes in his behaviour have been promised (her boyfriend never attends these meetings). Last week, when Helen declined to participate in an argument, Carol's boyfriend threatened her with physical violence. She contacted her on call manger, who organised for her to leave the house immediately and in safety. Because Carol was not able to look after Eleanor, Eleanor was admitted to hospital. Home care will not now be provided unless staff safety can be assured, and as the family are unable to manage, Eleanor will remain in hospital until a solution is found.

CONFIDENTIALITY

Confidentiality can be described as the nonoccurence of the unauthorised disclosure of information: in other words, where confidentiality is maintained, information is not disclosed without the explicit permission of the person or persons to whom it pertains.

Registered Nurses have a duty to respect the confidentiality of their clients (Nursing and Midwifery Council 2004). The European standards on privacy and confidentiality in healthcare state that individuals have a fundamental right to privacy and confidentiality and the right to control access to and disclosure of their health related information (McLelland 2006). The human right to self-determination also means that individuals have the right to decide who should or should not be given information about them. This right may, in exceptional cases (such as child protection issues), be overridden, as will be discussed in Chapter 9 (Dimond 2000). However, the usual principle is that information gained in the course of a relationship which develops because of a healthcare encounter should be treated as confidential. As well as being a professional requirement, maintaining confidentiality related to information about individuals and families is a part of demonstrating respect for them and is an important part of developing a trusting relationship (Johnson 2006).

As well as confidentiality related to healthcare information, such as diagnosis, treatment and care, all the information gleaned about an individual or family or their home in the course of healthcare work should remain confidential. By working in the home, staff are privy to privileged information regarding every aspect of a family's life. This may include: information about the family, their relationships, their home circumstances and environment, who visits them, their finances, and what telephone conversations they have. This should all be regarded as confidential, unless otherwise agreed, as it is only gained as a result of the healthcare relationship. Discussion of what may seem to be insignificant aspects of the family's life, circumstances, or situation, without the family's explicit consent, is usually inappropriate, breaches the requirements for confidentiality in professions and may be harmful for the child, young person, or their family.

It is expedient for staff to have absolute clarity over whom the child or young person and their family wish to have access to information, and what information they wish them to be given. This applies not only to health related information, but to other information gleaned in the course of working in the home. It may include apparently innocent information which is alluded to or requested in casual conversations with other visitors to the home or neighbours about aspects of family's life or house. However, if the information has been gleaned as a result of working in the family home, unless disclosure is agreed, this can constitute a breach of confidentiality and may provide information to individuals to whom the family do not wish to disclose it. This may be particularly challenging where parents or those with parental responsibility do not agree over disclosure of information. It requires staff to be clear over their responsibilities and to identify to children, young people, parents, and other family, friends or acquaintances what their boundaries are and why they may have to withhold information which may seem trivial.

Case study

Angela works with Jake's family. Jake's maternal grandmother lives nearby and often comes to visit. The family always seem very close to Jake's grandparents, and discuss what his aunts, uncles and other relations are doing. One afternoon, when Angela was at home with Jake his grandmother called in to visit, as she often does. She noticed a card on the shelf from Jake's uncle Joe and read this. She asked if Joe had been in contact, and whether he had had a good time, as the card was from a holiday in Spain. Angela said she thought he had phoned the previous night.

Angela later heard Hannah on the telephone to her mother saying that Jake's uncle was still away and that Angela must have been mistaken. It transpired that although Jake's uncle had returned to the UK his grandmother had been of the opinion that he was still away, as he had declined to attend a family event the coming weekend. Angela had disclosed information which she had only gleaned from overhearing a conversation in the course of her work, and had shared this with a person whom the family did not want to share it with.

SUMMARY

Working with families in their homes presents staff with some very specific challenges and considerations. Whilst some of these apply to all staff who work in the community setting, where staff are regular visitors in the family home, and spend many hours there, assisting parents in the day-to-day care of their child, there are additional considerations.

The issues that especially pertain to staff in this situation include negotiating the rules of what for families is their home but for staff is their workplace, what each party can reasonably expect from the other, and what part families want staff to play in their lives and homes as well as in meeting the child or young person's health related care. This may include how the family would like staff to be known to other children, friends, relations, and neighbours who may speak to them. It also requires clarity over the input that families want and staff will be able to provide to the child's siblings.

Staff who work closely with families in their homes have to negotiate the delicate balance between support and intrusion and be aware that, although families value the support they provide, in many cases they would ideally prefer to be able to care for their child without assistance. There are many factors that make it difficult for staff not to intrude on families' privacy, but thinking about how these can be minimised and being aware of the range of ways in which their presence can be an intrusion may enable staff to reduce these. Staff should also be aware of the need to take great care over confidentiality of information, not only related to the child or young person's health needs, but to all aspects of family life and information gained as a result of them being present in the family home.

Although families' rights and privacy should be a prime concern for staff, staff also have the right to safety and well-being at work. Whilst there are some differences in interpretation of the Health and Safety at work act when the workplace is a private home, staff should not tolerate or be expected to tolerate known risk to their personal safety and well-being.

Chapter 6
Supporting Young People

The number of children who have complex and continuing health needs, and the medical and technical developments which have enabled their life expectancy to be increased means that there is a growing population of young adults who have such needs (Department for Education and Skills and Department of Health 2006).

Whilst the principles of providing support at home described in the other chapters of this book apply to young people as well as to children and their families, there are some specific issues which those involved in supporting adolescents who have complex and continuing health needs should take into account. This chapter discusses some of these.

DEVELOPING INDEPENDENCE

Adolescence is often described as a time when young people are developing their independence. However, it is probably more accurate to describe it as a time when there is a significant change in the balance of independence or dependence which young people have on other individuals, such as their parents. Although the process of developing independence begins in infancy, it is more intense in adolescence. Young people are developing a strong sense of their own identity; exploring and discovering their personal values; acquiring the type of interpersonal skills they will need to function in adult relationships; negotiating a new relationship with their family; developing a degree of emotional, personal, and financial independence from their parents; and making plans for their future (Christie and Viner 2005; Turner 2006). The timing of the changes associated with the development of independence in adolescence varies from individual to individual, and also depends on the social and cultural expectations of the environment in which they live (Christie and Viner 2005).

The transition to independence requires young people who have complex health needs to accomplish the same developmental tasks and overcome the same challenges as other adolescents. However, they often face additional barriers which their peers do not. A major aspect of this may be that other people confuse their physical needs with their ability to be emotionally and cognitively independent (Department for Education and Skills and Department of Health 2006). An important part of young people who have complex health needs being enabled to achieve their optimum level of independence is others accepting their right to become independent. A person's health needs and the fact that they may be physically dependent on others does not reduce their right or ability to make choices about their lives. A young person being physically dependent on others or requiring some assistance with physical tasks should not be seen as meaning that they cannot be cognitively, emotionally and psychologically independent.

One of the challenges that their physical limitations may impose on young people is that, as Chapter 2 discusses, they may find it difficult to meet with their peers, and particularly to do so without an adult accompanying them. As well as limiting their social opportunities, having to be accompanied, and especially having to be accompanied by an adult, may mean that the young person feels less able to express and explore their thoughts and ideas than their peers do. Where they may, as a child, have been accompanied by a parent to social events or to play with other children, young people may prefer a person who is unrelated to them, or closer to their age, to be with them when they meet their peers. This may not create the constraints which a parent or other adult might on their contributions to peer interactions. Having a person close to their own age with them may enable young people to join in with their peers more easily and facilitate more natural interactions for the whole group.

Enabling young people who use specialised communication systems to develop independence, interact with their peers, and form social relationships may be especially challenging. They depend on people being prepared to take the time to listen carefully if their speech is difficult, to learn to use the method of communication which they use, or to speak considerately if their hearing is impaired. This potentially impedes their developing independence by reducing the number of their peers with whom they can talk and the number of people with whom they can speak one to one. It also often means that they cannot join in group discussions as easily or spontaneously as their peers can. This may limit their ability to openly discuss and explore their experiences and ideas and to chat informally with groups of their peers as other young people would.

Case study

Tamila is 17. She requires assistance with all her daily living needs, finds speech difficult and uses a communication aid. She attended mainstream school, and despite frequent episodes of illness and hospitalisation, gained good grades in her GCSEs. She has continued in the sixth form at school, and wants to go to university.

Recently, Tamila attended a family wedding. One person asked her mother, Ornella, what Tamila would be doing when she left school. They appeared very surprised when Ornella pointed to Tamila's communication aid and encouraged them to listen to what Tamila had to say about her future. They also seemed surprised that she was taking her A levels and planned to go to university. Ornella described how: 'They asked me later, "How will she manage at university? Is she really planning to go?" I said "She will manage the same way she does now. She will have a carer with her, who helps her with everything. We are planning for her to live away from home, like another girl of her age would. The university she wants to go to have already spoken to us, and we have talked about special accommodation. Her carers will be her arms and legs, like they are now. They will help her with all her physical tasks, and doing her washing, tidying the room she lives in, the practicalities of writing cheques and paying her bills, taking her to lectures, but she is a clever girl, and just because her body doesn't work well physically, why shouldn't she go to university?" She already manages her own money, the carers have to do tasks for her, but she plans it and budgets it herself. Of course it has all taken a long time to think about and organise, and she still has to get her grades, but it was as if they didn't think she should be able to live away from home, or study.'

Allowing a young person who has complex health needs to become independent may sometimes be particularly challenging for their parents. In most cases children who have complex health needs require a greater level of input from their parents over a longer period of time than other children. This can create a very different relationship to that which other children and their parents have and may make the young person realigning their level of dependence on their parents as they reach adolescence more difficult, physically and emotionally, for both parties.

Parents have usually developed expertise in their child's needs, and have become accustomed to being constantly vigilant and planning ahead of events to ensure their child's safety. Taking a step back from this and allowing anyone else, including the young person themselves, to take on such responsibility may be very difficult. Allowing a young person to become independent can be challenging for any parent. However, where parents have made decisions regarding health related quality of life, continuation and development of treatment and care in the past, handing such responsibility over to their child may be very difficult, especially when the young person's views are at odds with theirs. It may also be difficult to determine at what stage and in what circumstances the young person, rather than their parent, should make decisions. This is discussed in more detail in Chapter 8 in relation to children and young people's rights. However, the shifting of responsibility in adolescence may be a particularly challenging time for young people and their parents, and even more so where the young person has complex health needs.

In some cases, as well as having to consciously take a step back and enable their child to become independent, parents of young people with complex needs may have to encourage others to see their child as a young person who is entitled to independence. For example, they may have to encourage service providers to modify service provision to facilitate independence, and create opportunities for their child to become independent. Thus, whilst parents may find it difficult to allow their child to become independent, they may also have to take the lead in facilitating and encouraging others to facilitate their child's independence.

When information about a young person's health is being discussed, and decisions are being made, staff need to consider the young person's needs and rights together with the rights and responsibilities of their parents. They have to seek to avoid behaving in a way that fosters continued dependence by the young person, but which does not devalue parents' past and continued involvement in their child's life (Department for Education and Skills and Department of Health 2006). The transition to young people making their own decisions regarding their health, like all aspects of supporting young people through the transition from childhood to adulthood, should be a gradual process in which the young person and their parents feel supported and valued. Achieving this can be very difficult, and one of the skills required for working with young people and their families is the ability to work towards this balance.

RISK TAKING

Risk can be defined as 'a situation involving exposure to danger, the possibility that something unpleasant may happen' (Soanes et al. 2001). Risks exist because things that are considered to have value are placed in a situation in which they could be lost. In general, there is also some perceived potential gain for a risk to be worth taking. Risk taking behaviour is therefore the voluntary participation in activities or behaviours that contain, or are seen to contain, a significant degree of risk, along with the potential for some benefit.

Adolescence appears to be a time at which individuals are more likely to engage in risk taking behaviour than at other times. Many reasons for this have been suggested, including the differences between the physical changes of puberty, which impel adolescents toward seeking excitement, and the slower maturation of the cognitive-control system, which regulates these impulses, making adolescence a time of heightened vulnerability for risky behaviour (Reyna and Farley 2006; Steinberg 2007).

Risk taking in adolescence is often seen as a negative entity, for example being associated with substance abuse or reckless behaviour, with the gains often associated with peer acceptance. However, risk taking is an essential part of learning. A child has to take risks in order to progress in many areas of development, such as walking, talking, playing and developing friendships. By experiencing successes and failures, and then learning and adjusting their behaviour and expectations accordingly they learn (Stipek et al. 1992). Similarly, what might be defined as healthy risk taking is a positive tool in an adolescent's life for discovering, developing, and consolidating their identity, understanding how relationships work, and how they will be expected to function in the adult world. It is also important in the development of autonomy, and learning to take responsibility for one's own actions (Sharland 2006). Risk taking is therefore an essential part of the development of independence. It exists on a continuum, in which some risk taking is harmful whilst some is beneficial (Feldstein and Miller 2006; Sharland 2006).

Individuals place different values on a number of aspects of quality of life, and have different priorities and beliefs. As a result, individual attitudes to risk vary, including the relative value placed on what may be gained or lost. What one individual would see as healthy risk taking might be seen by another as reckless behaviour. Equally, one person might place a potential gain more highly than another, so that what in risk-benefit terms is a good or worthwhile risk to one person is an unnecessary or reckless risk to another. In adolescence, the counterpart of risk is often the gain of peer acceptance, which those outside adolescence may not value as highly as young people do.

Young people who have complex health needs may find risk taking more difficult than their peers. They are likely to have additional risks to take into account which their peers do not. For example, the risk involved in mixing alcohol and certain medication, the risk involved in not disclosing a medical condition versus the risk of their peers viewing them as different if they do disclose it (Hewitt-Taylor 2007). For their parents, the process of allowing or watching their child taking risks can be very difficult. The protection parents have had to provide for their child over many years, including protecting them from negative responses from other people, fighting for their place in society, services and even their right to life can make allowing them to take risks more difficult than it is for other parents.

Although it may be very difficult for parents, McConky and Smyth (2003) describe the importance of allowing and enabling young people who have complex needs to make decisions about risks and to take the risks which they see as appropriate. They describe how a 'danger-avoidance' strategy may restrict the young person's freedom of choice and autonomy and mean that they become lonely and isolated. Staff who work with young people who have complex health needs should aim to support them and their parents in a way that facilitates the development of independent risk taking.

Case study

Steven is 18. He has muscular dystrophy, uses a wheelchair, and requires CPAP at night. He goes to college and enjoys going out with his friends at weekends and in the evenings.

When Steven was 15, his family were involved in lengthy and emotionally draining discussions about the options for Steven's ongoing treatment and care. After a great deal of discussion, a decision was made, involving Steven, his parents and his healthcare team, that he should have CPAP at night. Since then, he has enjoyed a better quality of life, been less tired during the day, slept better, and had fewer chest infections.

Steven has recently begun to stay out late with his friends, often until midnight. His parents think he has started to smoke. His mother explains: 'I know that for all parents, they don't want their teenage son to smoke. At 18, I know, really, it's none of my business, but with Steven ... I know he has to be with his friends, that they are important to him, that he enjoys being with them, and he needs to be a normal 18 year old, but, at the same time, we had all the discussion about his lungs, how bad they are, and how he needs CPAP at night. If his lungs get any worse, then that will be it. We can see what a difference it made. He was ... well, we were looking at losing him. So it's hard, knowing what he is doing, and what that could do, but at the same time, wanting him to enjoy himself, and have friends and do things with them. When he stays out late at the pub, he doesn't start his CPAP until midnight or one o'clock, and he gets up at seven to go to college, and you wonder, doesn't he need it for longer, does he not need more rest? Shouldn't he be more careful? So, I find it hard, knowing I have to stop seeing him as a child, letting him make his choices, but ... those choices mean we could lose him. I know that could just be selfish, because it's his choice, and if being with his friends makes him happy, then, I don't want the years he has to be lonely and unhappy.'

Young people who have complex health needs may have very different experiences of risk taking from their peers. They may be unable to take risks as spontaneously as another young person would and may have to depend on others to facilitate their risk taking. This means that as well as losing spontaneity, their risk taking may be subject to uninvited comment and discussion in a way that their peers' is not. Some risks which they would themselves choose to take may be unavailable because the person who would have to assist them is not prepared to be involved. Having to negotiate risk taking with another person means that their 'success' or 'failure' in risky activities is known by another person in a way that it might not be for other young people. This risk may pertain not only to activities that are considered dangerous but to the risk associated with everyday events and rejection or acceptance in social situations.

Despite the need to facilitate young people's risk taking, it may present legal or ethical challenges for staff, for example if a young person requests assistance to obtain nonprescription drugs, or engage in under-age drinking. Those who work with young people need to be clear about what their legal and professional obligations are, their duty to the young person, their duty to the young persons' parents, and their own rights.

DEVELOPING PEER RELATIONSHIPS

Throughout childhood, acceptance by peers is important for children's well-being (Sunwolf and Leets 2004). The formation of peer relationships in adolescence is very important for all young people's well-being, and gives them the opportunity to socialise and develop the skills required to conduct adult relationships. Interactions with their peers enable adolescents to develop their communication skills, practice self-disclosure, explore their identity, pursue and develop their interests and abilities. Their peers can also provide young people with a chance to see and think about the strategies which others use to cope with a range of situations and to consider how effective these are (Better Health 2001).

Having the opportunity to develop peer relationships is as important for young people who have complex health needs as for any other adolescent, but it is often more difficult for them to achieve this (Department for Education and Skills and Department of Health 2006). As described in Chapter 2, there are many things which can make it difficult for young people who have complex health needs to meet and communicate with their peers. Where a young person relies on others to facilitate their meetings with peers and even their communication, the relationship which forms is not as easy as where they can meet alone, spontaneously, or when they can join in a discussion unaided.

As Chapter 2 describes, young people who have complex health needs may not be able to join in the full range of their peers' activities, and often find it difficult to be fully included in a group in the way that other adolescents are. This may sometimes be because the activities which their able-bodied peers engage in are not possible for them, but may also be because of a lack of physical access to venues which they could enjoy. This can mean that they are limited to only meeting other disabled people and thus have less choice in friendships and meet a less varied group of the population. Carer availability and funding can also affect their ability to meet their peers and to join in unplanned events. This should be considered in service planning and funding.

Case study

Darren is 15. He uses a wheelchair, and needs CPAP at night. He goes to a mainstream school, and has a group of friends there. His friends often go to the park on the way home, to sit and talk, play on skateboards and bikes. Darren cannot use a bike or skateboard, but likes to go along to be a part of the group. One of his friends pushes him home.

At weekends, his friends often go to the local leisure centre, which is about two miles from Darren's house. Darren would like to go along but the centre has no wheelchair access beyond the main foyer. The café has three small steps down to it. He can walk a few steps, with considerable assistance, but his parents cannot always take him, and his wheelchair and equipment is too bulky to fit into a friend's car. In addition, he can only really go if his mother or father is available to go with him, because although his friends will push his wheelchair, they are not able to assist him with other things, such as supporting him to walk a few steps or helping him to the toilet.

One of the nurses suggested that Darren try a group for young disabled people which is close to his home. He attended twice, but explains: 'It was OK, but I want to be with the people I go to school with, not other people. All my mates are together at weekends, and I want to be there, too, not with a different crowd of people.'

IMAGE AND IDENTITY

Self-image, which can be defined as: 'the idea which one has of one's abilities, appearance and personality' (Soanes et al. 2001), and self-concept (the ideas which one has about oneself) contribute to a person's self-esteem, which has been defined as 'confidence in one's own worth or attributes' (Soanes et al. 2001). These are important for all young people, and the development of a positive self-image and self-concept are developmental tasks that can be challenging for all adolescents. However, young people who have a chronic illness may find developing a positive self-esteem even more difficult than their peers because of the values that others place on them and the attitudes which society has to them (Christie and Viner 2005; Strandmark 2004). This applies equally, and perhaps even more so, to young people who have complex health needs.

Breakey (1997) identifies that society tends to be preoccupied with physical perfection, with anyone who deviates from this labelled as different and less worthy. If other people respond negatively to an individual because of their physical needs, the person may begin to view themselves negatively. If young people who have complex health needs compare their appearance and physical capability with those popularly portrayed in the media, where there are few high profile disabled individuals to be role models to them, they may perceive themselves as less acceptable than their able bodied peers (Breakey 1997).

As well as the way in which others respond to a person's physical appearance, the extent to which they are accepted and valued by others affects their self-esteem. As this and other chapters have identified, the way in which society as a whole responds to children and young people who have complex health needs is not always positive, and many facilities exclude, by nonprovision, those who have disabilities. This may suggest to individuals that they are not valued, are different and less worthy than their peers, all of which may contribute to the development of poor self-esteem. In addition, how their peers perceive and treat young people may cause them to feel devalued. Noyes (2006a) found that some young people who have complex health needs are aware of changes in how individuals view them as their health needs alter: for example, friends no longer visiting and feeling excluded from friendships as their needs increase. Whilst the responses of individuals cannot be altered by service providers, facilitating support in a way that encourages the continuation of peer contact may assist towards minimising this type of experience.

SEXUALITY AND SEXUAL EXPRESSION

The development of a sexual self is an integral part of the transition to adulthood (Earle 2001). Sexuality is an important part of everyday life for people in all societies, and contributes to one's identity and self-esteem (Godfrey 1999; Nye 1999). Therefore a holistic approach to providing support for young people who have complex health needs should include consideration of their sexuality. It has been suggested that people are only given their full respect as people when their sexuality is seen as a vital component of their humanity (McCann 2000). A part of respecting young people is therefore acknowledging their sexual needs. However, there is a suggestion that disabled young people and adults do not have the opportunities for sexual expression and exploration that their nondisabled peers have (Earle 1999).

Many of the problems that young people who have complex health needs face in relation to their sexual needs are associated with the perceptions others have of them. For example, Potgieter and Gadija (2005) found that the opportunities which adolescents with spinal injuries have to express their sexuality is affected more by the attitudes of others than the limitations imposed by their physical disabilities. Shakespeare (1999) describes how people with impairments are often, albeit possibly subconsciously, regarded by society as belonging to a third, asexual, gender and are therefore not expected to have sexual needs. Furthermore, it has been suggested that disabled people are generally infantilised by society, and as such consideration of their sexuality is seen as inappropriate, and disabled people perceived as abnormal when they express an interest in sexual exploration and sexual expression (Earle 2001).

The opportunities that young people who have complex health needs have for sexual expression may also be affected by them continuing to need to live at home and being dependent on their families at a time when other young people would live away from home and be independent of their parents. This may reduce the privacy which they have to express sexual feelings and to engage in sexual relationships (Sakellariou and Algado 2006). In addition, their physical limitations may mean that they require assistance to be involved in sexual activities and it may be difficult for young people to ask for such assistance, and those supporting them may be unwilling to offer to help them.

The assistance that these young people require to explore their sexuality may include help with a range of activities associated with sexual need: the provision of accessible information and advice; assistance to attend social events; and assistance to experience sexual activity (Earle 1999). However, society's attitudes to sexual activity generally and to disabled people having a sexual self may mean that assisting young people to explore their sexual needs is not seen as important or even appropriate. In addition, the values and beliefs of the disabled person may differ from those of the person who is asked to assist them. This makes young people being able to explore their sexual self more problematic than their peers, who would engage in whatever activity they have decided is appropriate, without requiring the approval or co-operation of an additional person.

All individuals who have disabilities may encounter difficulties when they seek assistance in expressing their sexual needs. However, because a number of the challenges which they face relate to the attitudes and values of others, this is likely to be even more problematic when their sexual needs are not in line with what society holds to be conventional sexual behaviour (Earle 1999). For example, gay, lesbian and bisexual people with disabilities may face particular barriers to exploring their sexuality and having their sexual needs met (Abbott and Howarth 2007).

Young people who have complex health needs may experience difficulty in obtaining information and services on reproductive and sexual health. A survey of family planning services in Northern Ireland identified that physical access to these clinics was incomplete, so that disabled young people did not have the opportunity to use the services that their nondisabled peers could (Anderson and Kitchin 2000). The Disability Discrimination Act (HMSO 2005) means that access to such services should now be equally available to disabled people. However, a further issue is that young people who depend on others to enable them to access services and to communicate may have to negotiate accessing services with another person, or discuss intimate matters with a third party present, which they may find intimidating and intrusive.

The quality and relevance of the advice and information that is available to young people who have complex health needs may also be problematic. Many disabled people report not being able to obtain satisfactory professional advice about the impact of their impairments on their sexual health (Seymour 1998). There is some evidence that the information and advice available to disabled people often deals predominantly with problems of obtaining and maintaining erections, ejaculation and fertility for men, whilst women's sexuality is either ignored or reduced to concerns about fertility and motherhood (Earle 1999).

Case study

Tamila wants to discuss sexual health issues with someone. Although she can join in discussions with her peers about sex and sexuality, she feels that there are specific matters about which she would like advice, because of her disability. These include physical aspects of her disability, advice on contraception and other advice such as what activities she can reasonably expect her carers to be involved in assisting her with, should she develop a sexual relationship.

She has tried looking for information on the internet, but this is very limited and tends to focus on developing friendships and personal relationships, not information on sexual relationships.

Tamila has not found anyone who she feels will be able to answer all her questions, but thought that the family planning service might be useful and point her in the right direction for other services. However, her carer finishes work as soon as the school day ends, and she does not want to ask her mother or brother, who otherwise assist her, to accompany her.

She eventually persuaded a friend to accompany her. However, they arrived at the family planning clinic and found that, although the interior was all on one level, there were seven steps up to the door, and the ramp was unavailable due to maintenance work. Tamila was therefore not able to keep her appointment.

Disabled people are more likely to experience physical, sexual and emotional abuse than any other group (Cambridge 1999; Bernard 1999). They are more likely to rely on others for all, or some, of their care and this dependency creates an opportunity for abuse and an environment in which the risk of abuse is increased (Bernard 1999). Severely disabled people and those with communication difficulties may also find it difficult to articulate their abuse, and may be less likely than other people to be believed (Sant Angelo 2000). The abuse of disabled people is a serious problem, but whilst disabled people have the right to be protected from sexual abuse and exploitation, concern with this risk should not be used to deny disabled people their sexual identity. Just as the labelling of disabled people as asexual is inappropriate, so too is an atmosphere in which any evidence of sexuality or discussion thereof is taboo. Such an atmosphere only serves to quash a person's sexual needs and may, in fact, serve to increase the incidence, or worsen the experience, of sexual abuse.

FURTHER EDUCATION

Accessing further education and employment opportunities presents a greater challenge for young people who have complex health needs than it does for other young people (Department for Education and Skills and Department of Health 2006).

There are a comparative lack of post compulsory education and training opportunities for young people with complex health needs (Beresford 2004; Millar and Aitken 2005). Colleges may find it hard to support young people who use specialised communication systems, and where students need assistance with personal care, facilities for them may be lacking (Millar and Aitken 2005). It is often difficult for young people to obtain information regarding college places and young people who have complex health needs often encounter lengthy processes in seeking and obtaining funding for post compulsory education (Millar and Aitken 2005). The provision of appropriate transport may also be problematic, and may be exacerbated by the paucity of colleges that can cater for young people needs, making lengthy journeys a commonplace necessity. The planning involved in a young person's transition to a College of Further Education should include how all aspects of support (including funding, equipment and personnel) can be facilitated (Burchardt 2005).

Case study

Darren wants to continue his studies after school, but there are very few colleges that are able to cater for his needs. He and his parents began looking for a college which would be suitable for him when he was 14.

Darren eventually gained a place at a specialist college for young people with physical disabilities. However, during his final term at school he was advised that transport to the college, which is 20 miles from his home, would not be funded. This means that his mother will have to find a way of getting Darren and his carer to and from college every day, and funding this. They have appealed the decision, and this is being considered at the end of July. Darren's college place starts on 3rd September.

Some children who have been in small classes at a specialist school, or have had one-to-one assistance may find making the transition to a college environment difficult. For example, classes may be larger, the total number of students considerably greater, the level of assistance reduced and the environment more impersonal (Hewitt-Taylor 2007). It may be helpful for transition planning for young people who have complex health needs to include a way for those who wish to attend large mainstream colleges but have been used to a smaller, more personalised environment, to be enabled in this process by a controlled decrease in the support provided. As well as immediate post-16 education, there should be opportunities for disabled people to return to education throughout their lives, as other people can, and for this to encompass the same range of experiences and qualifications that their peers can access (Burchardt 2005). This should also apply to those who have complex health needs, and service provision should take this into account.

PREPARING FOR EMPLOYMENT

Gaining employment is almost certainly more of a challenge for young people who have complex and continuing health needs than it is for other young people (Department For Eductaion and Skills and Department of Health 2006). There is relatively little evidence about the employment of young people who have complex health needs. However, disabled young people in general do not enjoy equal employment status with their nondisabled peers and face many barriers to taking up employment (Thornton 2003). Approximately 85 per cent of nondisabled people are in employment compared with 40–50 per cent of disabled people, with employment rates being lower for disabled women than for men. Disabled people are twice as likely as nondisabled people to have no qualifications, and unqualified nondisabled people are almost three times as likely to be in employment as their disabled counterparts. The employment gap narrows, but remains, for disabled people with higher levels of qualification (Thornton 2003). It is likely that this difference applies equally, if not more so, to young people who have complex health needs.

Although there is evidence that young disabled people fare less well in the employment market than their peers, this does not appear to be because of them lacking aspiration or initial motivation to gain employment. Burchardt (2005) found that the scope and level of the work related hopes and aims of disabled 16-year-olds were similar to those of their nondisabled peers. However, the experiences of disabled and nondisabled young people diverges sharply after they leave school. At the age of 26, disabled people were nearly four times as likely to be unemployed or involuntarily out of work than nondisabled people. The occupational outcomes of 39% of disabled people were below the level to which they had aspired 10 years previously, compared with 28% of nondisabled people. Those who were in employment had earnings that were 11% lower than those of their nondisabled counterparts who had the same level of educational qualification. This lack of actual equality of employment opportunity can make it very hard for disabled young people to sustain their initial high aspirations, and can not only affect their employment but their self-esteem and feelings of worth and well-being.

Thornton (2003) identifies that young people who have disabilities need more personalised, intensive and flexible support than is currently provided to enable them to gain more equal access to the employment market. This may include providing them with much more support in entering employment, including facilitating work placements related to their interests (Burchardt 2005). Service provision for young people who have complex health needs should also take into account how they will be supported to seek and obtain employment, with support being made available for work placements, preparation of applications, and interviews. There also needs to be clarity over the support which will be available for them should they be successful in job applications so that they can confidently assure potential employers of their ability to fulfil their roles.

TRANSITION TO ADULT SERVICES

Transition from children's to adult services can be defined as:

> A purposeful planned process that addresses the medical, psychosocial, educational and vocational needs of adolescents and young adults with chronic physical and medical conditions as they move from child centered to adult orientated healthcare systems (Department for Education and Skills and Department of Health 2006)

Planning that includes all the relevant agencies and centres on the hopes, aspirations, education, training and employment needs of young people is the hallmark of good transition planning (Department for Education and Skills and Department of Health 2006). Local agencies are required to have a system of person-centred planning for all young people moving from children's to adult services and to provide effective links between children's and adult services in both health and social care (Department of Health 2001a). However, there is still often poor co-ordination between services and a lack of involvement of the young person themselves in the transition to adult services. Some young people are transferred without adequate planning and with inadequate care plans. This can mean that they do not have access to the full range of adult services they need, and in some instances adult services may not have the type of provision required for young people who have complex health needs (Beresford 2004; Department for Education and Skills and Department of Health 2006). This may mean that they experience a reduction in services when child care services cease to provide for them (Beresford 2004).

Improving the transition to adult services and subsequent provision within adult services for young people who have complex health needs requires time, resources and commitment. However, the cost of these is minor compared with what has been invested in them during childhood and the cost of their future care and input, which is likely to be more easily and more effectively managed if their transition is well planned (Department for Education and Skills and Department of Health 2006). As the number of young people who have complex health needs increases, service provision will need to develop to meet their needs at the time of transition.

Although transition to adult services is an important time, which requires carefully planned input, there is no one right time or age for transition to occur, and rigid rules on this are usually unhelpful. The right timing depends, amongst other things, on the developmental readiness and health status of each person. Transition may occur because it is thought that the individuals' need would be better met in adult services, because the person has statutorily become an adult, or because they appear ready to move on (Beresford 2004). However, it should be a joint decision between service providers, young people and their families that the time to commence the preparation for moving to adult services is right. Trust policies and commissioning processes should facilitate this degree of flexibility and person centredness.

Transition to adult services should be a process, not a single event (Department for Education and Skills and Department of Health 2006). Ideally, it should be planned well before the person leaves children's services as an effective transition can require a great deal of investigation, co-ordination and negotiation. This includes: identifying interested and capable adult services, deciding how the processes of information transfer will happen, negotiating administrative support, and ensuring the involvement of primary care, education and social care. For the young person, it is important that they have a trusted adult who can challenge and support them at this time, act as an advocate and assist them to develop self-advocacy skills so that at the time of transition and beyond their needs are stated, heard and acted on (Department for Education and Skills and Department of Health 2006).

Communication is in many respects the most important issue in effecting a smooth transition from children's to adult services (Department for Education and Skills and Department of Health 2006). The number of communications required for this process means that having one key point of reference for young people and their families, but also for all services, is essential. The Key Worker and Lead Professional are vital parts of the transition process, to provide one known, clear point of contact for all the parties involved.

There are many models of transition, and the best approach to this process depends on the individual child and family and the resources that are available. Some areas use a dedicated follow-up service in the adult setting for young people, with no other direct input from children's services once transition occurs. This may be the simplest model, but to be effective it requires good co-ordination between the children's and adult services at the time of transfer (Department for Education and Skills and Department of Health 2006).

An alternative approach is the provision of a seamless clinic, which begins in childhood or adolescence and continues into adulthood, with professionals from children's and adult services providing ongoing care as appropriate. This approach allows the young person to continue to benefit from the input of specialists from children's services, and from those who are able to provide for appropriate management of adult issues. It allows both groups of specialists to learn from one another and from the young person and their family. There will still be the question of when children's services cease to be involved with any individual, but this approach allows a more gradual phasing out of input from children's services and tailoring transition to individual need (Department for Education and Skills and Department of Health 2006).

Another option is lifelong follow-up in the child health setting, an approach which sometimes happens by default, where no other options exist and adult services are not set up to meet the young person's needs. This ensures continuity, but may make it more difficult for the child to access expertise on adult issues such as sexual health, vocational and benefits issues (Department for Education and Skills and Department of Health 2006). It may also detract from the young person being seen as an adult, and developing independence.

In other situations, a generic transition team may exist, where dedicated nurse specialists ensure that all young people who have complex health needs go through appropriate transition in all aspects of service provision. In other cases, transition co-ordinators who work with children and young people who have rare conditions cover a wide geographical area and ensure that they access all the appropriate services at the time of transition (Department for Education and Skills and Department of Health 2006).

Whichever model is used, the mainstay of good transition planning is that it should be person centred, and that clear communication and planning between services occurs (Department for Education and Skills and Department of Health 2006).

SUMMARY

An increasing number of children who have complex and continuing health needs are now living into adulthood. This means that there is a developing population of adolescents who have this type of health need. Although many of the principles that underpin providing effective support for all children and their families apply equally to young people, there are some specific issues which staff who work with adolescents who have complex and continuing health needs have to consider.

Young people who have complex and continuing health needs may find the transition to independence much more difficult than their peers, because of their needs, and the way in which these are provided for, but also because of the attitudes which society has to them. They may face many barriers to developing peer relationship, engaging in leisure activities and taking risks. They are also likely to find it more difficult to access further education and to gain employment than their peers. The sexual needs of disabled people are generally poorly recognised and provided for, and this applies equally, and possibly more, to young people who have complex health needs.

Service provision for young adults who have complex health needs is likely to be best facilitated if an effective transition to adult services can be achieved. This usually requires advanced and diligent planning, and a Key Worker or Lead Professional who can co-ordinate this process and work closely with the young person to ensure that their voice is heard, listened to, and acted on.

Chapter 7
Grief, Loss and Bereavement

Loss concerns a situation where an individual no longer has something, or has less of something. Everyone will, during their lifetime, experience loss of some kind, but what constitutes a loss and the significance of this differs from person to person, depending on many things, including the value that they attached to what is lost, and the impact of the loss on other aspects of their life.

Grief can be described as a feeling of intense sorrow (Soanes et al. 2001). Grief is something that all people will experience, and, like loss, grief can be felt because of a wide range of events, and whether a specific circumstance or event causes an individual to grieve, the severity of that grief and how it is managed varies from individual to individual. Whilst grief is a painful experience, it also has the potential to enable individuals to experience personal growth (Murray 2000). Grief is often can be caused by loss and to grieve is a normal human response to loss (Murray 2000).

Bereavement refers to being deprived of someone through death (Soanes et al. 2001) and is therefore a very specific form of loss and linked with the experiences and feelings of loss and grief.

Grief, loss and bereavement are almost universal experiences, and ones with which all healthcare staff deal in their personal lives and in their work. However, there are some specific aspects of grief, loss and bereavement which those supporting children and young people who have complex and continuing health needs and their families should consider. This chapter discusses some of these issues.

GRIEF AND LOSS FOR CHILDREN AND YOUNG PEOPLE

Like everyone, children and young people who have complex and continuing health needs may experience loss and grief related to a variety of life events. The cause, intensity, timing and duration of their feelings will be as individual for them as they are for anyone else. It may be tempting to assume that the major losses which they feel relate to their health needs, but children and young people who have complex health needs are also likely to suffer losses that are unrelated to their health condition, in the same way that their peers do.

Children and young people feel the pain of loss as intensely as adults do (Riley 2003). Whilst it may not always be clear what an individual child or young person's level of understanding is, the assumption should be that all individuals, regardless of their health needs or perceived cognitive level, feel loss. As previous chapters have identified, a person's ability to express themselves verbally should not be confused with their ability to experience emotions, and this applies equally to feelings of loss and grief. However, if a child or young person has difficulty in communicating, they may have difficulty in expressing their feelings or finding someone who is willing and able to facilitate them explaining and exploring their feelings as another person would. Those who support children and young people who have altered communication methods need to allow them the chance to express and discuss their feelings related to loss, and be alert to other clues which may indicate how they are feeling.

Whilst no assumptions should be made about what loss means to or for any individual, it may be useful to consider possible sources of loss for children and young people who have complex health needs. This may assist staff to identify situations where loss or grief may be felt, and, especially where additional communication skills are needed, enable them to be more alert to possible cues that the person whom they are supporting is experiencing feelings of loss or grief.

Case study

Tanya is seven. She has always been dependent on others to assist her in all her daily activities, has very limited speech and finds using a communication aid difficult. She has recently learned that she will be having surgery to have a gastrostomy performed and will subsequently be fed via the gastrostomy. She is not happy about having to go to hospital and have surgery, however what she is very upset about is that she feels she will not be a part of family mealtimes anymore and will not eat with her peers at school. She thinks this will make her even more different from her classmates, and that she will miss out on events with her family and peers even more than she does now.

It is very difficult for Tanya to explain how she feels. People have been very good at explaining to her what will happen when she goes to hospital, and what her gastrostomy looks like and will do. However, she has not been able to tell anyone how she feels about the impact that a gastrostomy will have on her life. She has started to cry at mealtimes, to try to let people know her feelings, but people tend to misinterpret this as her being upset at having difficulty eating, and think that it shows that her having a gastrostomy will be a good thing. Her mother thinks that she is unhappy about the idea of her gastrostomy, but everyone else is convinced, and trying to convince her, her that she is wrong.

Children and young people may always have had complex health needs, or may experience a sudden and unexpected change in their situation, health and abilities. In the former case they may feel the loss of opportunity for things which they will never have or experience, and in the latter they may grieve the loss of what they no longer have. A child or young person who is aware that they have different abilities to their peers may feel grief at their inability to do what other children and young people of their age can. This may be high-lighted when their peers achieve certain milestones or when younger siblings develop skills that they will never attain. They may lose social opportunities, education opportunities, and the hopes they had for their career, or may be aware that their opportunities are different from those of their peers. They may lose their expected future roles, anticipated achievements, relationships and independence and may also feel the injustice of their position. As iden-tified in Chapter 6, young people who have complex health needs may not have lesser aspirations than their peers, but may discover that they have less opportunities.

Children or young people whose health is deteriorating may grieve for their increasing loss of functional ability and may be aware that they are treated differently from the way they used to be. For example, Noyes (2006a) describes how some children who are dependent on mechanical ventila-tion notice that friends withdraw from them as their condition deteriorates. They may also be aware that they will die, or that their condition and abilities will deteriorate and may experience anticipatory grief related to this.

The range of events or situations which may cause children and young people to feel loss, and the number of occasions on which they are exposed to such experiences can mean that they experience what has been termed 'chronic sorrow'. Here one loss is followed by another, sometimes in different areas of life or related to different aspects of life. The consequence is that the individual does not have any significant period of time in which they are not having to adapt to loss and address feelings of grief (Eakes et al. 1998; Scornaienchi 2003).

Case study

Nathan is 14. He has muscular dystrophy. His younger brother, Ewan, is 12. Nathan is gradually becoming less able, and now spends most of his day in a wheelchair. Nathan recalls his brother learning to walk, and teaching him to kick a football. His younger brother is now an excellent footballer, plays cricket, loves riding a bike and skateboarding, whilst Nathan is becoming steadily less able. His younger brother goes out alone with his friends, while he has to rely on an adult or his younger brother coming with him to assist him. As his younger brother becomes more independent, Nathan feel that he is becoming more dependent. He is aware that as his brother plans for his future, his own future is diminishing. His physical health is deteriorating, he has less energy to devote to his school work and leisure activities. He knows that he is unlikely to live for many years longer, so his plans for further education and employment are receding in relevance. As his peers discuss what they plan to do next, and his younger brother discusses his hopes and dreams, he feels that none of this applies to him. He feels the loss of his future, but also how this impacts on his present as he has lost so much of what he might have had in common with his peers.

Although some aspects of loss may relate to the child or young persons' health needs, in many cases the way in which they are treated and catered for by society, rather than their physical disability per se, causes or creates feelings of loss or grief (Green 2007). The way in which children and young people are perceived by others, the responses they receive, and the manner in which they are spoken to, included, and consulted may be different from that which they see their peers experiencing, or may change as their health needs change. The facilities that are available to them, their degree of privacy and the respect they are afforded may alter, and the expectations which people have of them, not only physically but also cognitively and socially may change. If they have difficulty in speaking, they may feel that their altered ability to communicate and the way in which this changes how other people view them. This may include the difference in the way and extent to which people seek to engage with them, and how far they are perceived as able to communicate.

Case study

Noah is 10. When he was seven he was involved in a road traffic accident and sustained a high spinal injury, which has left him dependent on others for his physical needs. Noah misses playing football with his friends, he misses riding his bike, and

> being able to choose what he does, without asking anyone. He misses playing on his own, being able to move his toys around, and being able to read on his own, because someone now has to help him choose a book and turn the pages for him.
>   Noah describes how people speak to him differently now from how they did before his accident. He explains: 'When I was seven, before the car crash, people would ask me what I liked to do, what I liked playing with, what I was doing at school, what I wanted to be when I grew up. Now I'm ten, and they don't. They ask my Mum.'

As well as grief related to their own condition, children who have complex health needs may experience loss if someone whom they know dies or has a significant change in their condition. This may be another child at their school, at a group that they attend, a sibling who is older than them and has a similar disorder to them, or a family member or friend who has no health needs like their own. Their grief may include loss of the individual, but, where the person had a similar condition to theirs, may also include an element of anticipatory grief, and heightening of concerns about their own illness and mortality.

SOURCES OF LOSS FOR PARENTS

Parents whose children have complex and continuing health needs may experience loss for a variety of reasons. Parenthood has increasingly become a planned, personal and emotional investment, often in a single child (Krueger 2006). Where a child is not 'as planned' this can be a source of loss and grief for their parents as they lose the child whom they had planned, and planned for.

The losses parents experience, like those of children and young people, will be highly individual, and no assumptions should be made about these. However, they may lose many of the experiences they expected to have as parents (Barr and Millar 2003). This can begin with antenatal events, such as a high-risk pregnancy changing the pregnancy and planning for their baby which they anticipated. If a baby is born prematurely, or is unwell after being born, the time after their birth is often very different from that for which parents had planned. This can include changes to expected and planned for activities, such a feeding the baby, bathing them, what they will be dressed in, and taking the baby home. A newborn baby being identified as disabled or at risk of disability may mean that their parents cannot enjoy their baby as other parents can and have concerns and anxieties which other parents do not about their future. In addition, as discussed in Chapter 3, the usual social markers which accompany a baby's birth may be lost and the expected celebration and congratulations be replaced by withdrawal, awkwardness or sympathy. The baby's homecoming may be delayed for many months and the baby may be unable to occupy the room or use the furniture which their parents had chosen, and the clothes and toys they had purchased for them. Their plans to attend parent and baby groups or activities with friends may also be changed.

There is also a great potential for parents to experience ongoing and renewed feelings of loss as their child grows up, especially at specific transition points in a child's life, or when their peers attain certain goals or milestones (Riesz 2004). As their child grows older, parents may feel the changes in the developmental milestones which their child achieves, and the contrast between their expectations for the activities which they can enjoy with them, and the activities which they can actually enjoy together. Parents whose children have complex health needs may also lose their expected involvement in their child's schooling. Whilst their input into their child and their education may be immense, they may not have the relationships they had expected with their child's teachers and other parents. If their child uses specialist transport to get to school they may not meet school staff and other parents as they would in other circumstances (Hewitt-Taylor 2007). They may also lose their plans and ambitions for their child's education and employment.

Case study

Frances recalls that: 'We had intended to have Greg at home, and the midwives were all very excited about that, and we were very excited too. They made this big thing of natural delivery, and home birth. Then of course Greg started dropping his heartbeat, and we had to go in, and then he lost his heartbeat altogether, and they had to do an emergency Caesarian. I felt really sad at the time, because the midwives had really talked up not having interventions, and we had everything planned at home. Then of course we were in hospital for 10 days. So, right from the start I didn't feel like things were how I expected. Then I struggled with feeding him. I did breast feed him, for six months, and it was struggle. But then you are so sold this idea that this is right, the best thing, and we had had so much else I felt hadn't gone to plan, so I was determined. I did ask even then, because I was sure something was wrong, but the midwife just said I was anxious, and had to relax. Really, it was as if it was my fault. So I suppose I feel I lost that as well, that idyllic picture of feeding your baby and enjoying it. Enjoying him. I always knew something had gone wrong, so from the very start, I could never relax, I was worried about him from day one.'

If families need assistance to care for their child, they may lose a great deal of their privacy, as described in Chapters 4 and 5. Their child's needs may mean that they lose personal time, and may have to radically alter their home environment. As well as the intrusion that this occasions, having medical equipment and staff in their home has been described by some mothers as a source of sorrow and pain, a constant reminder of the differences between them and other families (Wilson et al. 1998). As well as loss related to their child, parents whose children have complex health needs may lose elements of their own lives which have been important to them (Barr and Millar 2003). This may include employment, relationships, and financial security. They may need to review their priorities, life plans and lifestyle. Thus, parents may feel loss related to their child, and their life, but also loss related to their own lives, because of their child's needs and how these are provided for.

Green (2002) describes the very specific type of loss which parents whose child has a disability can experience, because the object of loss is still a very real and important presence in their lives. Although the child is still with their parents, and usually loved and valued for who they are, the expected and imagined narrative of their own life, their child's life and their future with their child is lost. Whilst this may not diminish the love parents feel for the child whom they have, the loss is still felt. In addition, the loss is ongoing. Not only must parents create a new narrative for themselves and their child, but, because of the often uncertain trajectory of complex health needs, this may have to be continually altered.

As well as altering the expected narrative for a particular child, if the child has a genetic disorder, this may also mean that parents' expectations for future children are altered. If the child's care needs are significant, this too may mean that plans for other children have to be modified.

Case study

Jane and Kieran have a three-year-old daughter, Faith, who has Spinal Muscular Atrophy Type 1. Jane explains: 'Faith is a gorgeous little girl. She is so loving, but as much as we love her, you do feel sometimes . . . my friends were all talking about first steps, and I just sat there thinking: "Faith won't be doing any of that." They are talking about getting rid of the buggy and I'm talking about getting a wheelchair. So, much as I love Faith, sometimes I do feel sad, that we didn't have any of that. Any of the things we expected to have. We didn't have any specific plans, because we are of the opinion you don't plan for your child, but you do still expect things, like that you'll go and play in the park, and buy them a trike. We were planning to have two, at least, but now we won't. So, in that way we lost another child as well.

My friends talk about their plans for their children, plans for the next one, plans for school and later. Well, our plans for Faith are that we will love her and care for her and make sure we all enjoy the time we have together. That's our plans. We plan what is best for her, and we plan . . . we do have to plan what will happen as she gets less able. We have had to make decisions about how much treatment we want for her. We have to plan, or not really plan, but we do know that she will not live long, and we won't have other children. So, our plans are very different form our friends.'

Parents, like children, may experience multifaceted losses which create feelings of chronic sorrow, where loss in relation to one aspect of life is followed by loss in another area. Thus, individuals may be trying to adjust to different aspects of their changed lives at the same time, or as they begin to adjust to one loss, another change or loss confronts them (Eakes et al. 1998; Scornaienchi 2003). For example, parents may have adapted to the need for their child to have long-term assisted ventilation, but if there is a problem with the child accessing education they may again experience loss associated with this new problem.

Some events may cause parents a complex mixture of grief and relief. For example, where a child has experienced a long and difficult diagnostic pathway, or if their parents have had fears or doubts about their health, their eventual diagnosis may be something of a relief, despite the loss associated with the finality of a diagnosis (Nuutila and Salantera 2005). This may represent loss of accumulation of hope that the child would improve, but a diagnosis may also be reassuring, as a named or known problem has been identified and the way in which this should be treated or managed is clearer and support may in some cases be more accessible (Hewitt-Taylor 2007).

Case study

Greg was described as a 'bit awkward' at his six-week check. He was behind in his motor developmental milestones, and became increasingly so. His parents took him to the GP on a number of occasions, but were always reassured that he was just a little slow and would catch up. He was seen by a physiotherapist, and made some progress in walking, but never walked unaided.

Eventually, when Greg was three, he was diagnosed as having cerebral palsy. Frances, explains: 'I was kind of relieved, in a way, because we knew what we were dealing with. We had always known there was a problem. I had known from when he was about a week old, even earlier. I just knew. On the one hand, I would have liked to be proved wrong. No one wants their child to have something wrong with them, but because I knew there was a problem, I was relieved in a way that we knew what it was, so we could do the right things for him. On the other hand, I was still hoping, even though I knew, all these years, I was hoping I was wrong. So my tiny hope, that everything was OK, was gone. That sick in your stomach feeling that, yes, I was right. This is it.'

In addition to loss of their own plans and expectations, parents may experience feelings of grief related to how society places and responds to them and their children (Green 2007). Seeing society's responses to their child, the sadness which this causes them and their child, and seeing their child cope with teasing, or stigmatisation can be a source of profound grief for parents.

Parent's loss and grief may also have an element of anticipatory grieving, as they are often aware of the frailty of their children's lives. This can be highlighted by the deterioration or death of peer or classmate with a similar disability. Like children, parents may grieve for the child and family concerned, but also because of the implications which this has for their own child (Judson 2004).

If a child dies, as well as loss of the child, parents may lose a significant and often overwhelming part of their own identity, especially if they have cared for their child for many years. Wood and Milo (2001) describe the loss of firstly having a child who has a disability, and then the loss which comes with their death. This may mean that the parents of a child with complex health needs may have an even greater grief load than parents whose child dies without a preceding long-standing illness. Assumptions should not be made regarding what a child and their needs mean for any person or family. As Chapter 3 discusses in more detail, there is great potential for healthcare professionals to underestimate the value which a child who has complex needs has for their parents. Green (2007) identifies that the exhaustion and challenges created by the practical tasks and societal barriers which parents face should not be confused with them feeling grief over the child as a person. For parents, losing a child who has complex health needs still means losing their child.

Case study

Nathan's mother, Joyce, knows another two boys who have muscular dystrophy. They have formed a small informal support group. One of the boys, Harry, was diagnosed as having muscular dystrophy at around the same time as Nathan, and was a year older than him. He recently developed a chest infection, from which he did not recover. Joyce explains:

'All the time Harry was in hospital I was praying he would get better. Mostly because he is a lovely boy, and his family and us are so close, but a part of me was like: "Don't let Harry die, because Nathan has the same thing, and he is only a year younger . . ." Ever since Harry went, I have been so afraid for Nathan. Every little thing, I think "Is this it?" Sometimes I have found it hard, physically exhausting, to look after Nathan, but now, I treasure everything I do for him, because I think: "How long have I got him for? Not long." And I can't bear that thought. Everyone thinks: "Well, she's had 10 years to get used to it. She knows what he's got." You never get used to the idea that your baby will die. Never.'

SOURCES OF LOSS FOR OTHER FAMILY MEMBERS

A child having complex health needs can mean that many members of their family experience feelings of loss or grief (Gilroy and Johnson 2004). This includes their siblings and other family members such as grandparents, aunts, and uncles.

If a child's brother or sister is unwell immediately after they are born, they may feel the loss of their promised brother or sister. If they have been jealous of or unhappy about the idea of having a brother or sister they may feel guilty and perceive that they caused their sibling to be sick or disabled. If a child develops complex health needs, their siblings may feel the loss of the brother or sister they had, and loss of the things which they used to do with them, or had hoped to do with them. This may not mean that they devalue or do not love the sibling whom they have, but grieve or feel loss for the one whom they expected, or the hopes, dreams or expectations which they had for their life with them.

As Chapter 3 describes, children may also lose tangible aspects of their own life if their brother or sister has complex health needs. This may include their free time being reduced, their social opportunities being changed, and their family's previous lifestyle altering (including changes in family holidays, outings, activities and housing). Siblings may also have less of their parents' time or attention, either because the focus is on the sick child, and the time taken for their care leaves little time for other things, or because the parents are themselves suffering loss and cannot focus easily on the needs of their other children. From the child's perspective, they may feel that their parents, as well as their sibling, have changed or been lost, and that their parents no longer love them, or no longer love them as much as they once did (Saldinger et al. 1999).

Like the child or young person and their parents, other children in the family may feel loss associated with other people's responses to their brother or sister. This may include them not being asked about their newborn brother or sister as other children are, children avoiding their sibling, or not including them in invitations as other siblings are. Siblings may also feel loss on behalf of their brother or sister, and see the injustice of society's responses to them and the opportunities which they do not have.

When a child dies, as well as missing their brother or sister, other children in the family may feel guilty about their death, especially if they have resented them, or felt aggrieved at the attention that their sibling received, and the changes in their own life that their sibling's needs occasioned. They may also feel that it is a punishment to them, or caused by them because of negative feelings towards their sibling (Gilroy and Johnson 2004).

Any family member may experience feelings of grief and loss related to a child or young person's complex health needs. This includes grandparents, aunts and uncles who may feel the loss of the child whom they expected, or the child whom they once knew, loss of the expectations which they had for that child and their role in their life. Like parents and siblings, they may feel sadness at how they see other people respond to and treat the child and the losses and struggles which they see them experience because of society's attitudes to them. In addition, they may feel grief and pain for the loss and grief which they see the child's parents experiencing.

THEORIES OF GRIEF, LOSS AND BEREAVEMENT

Although grief is a universal experience, it is also a very individual experience (Krueger 2006). People all have their own beliefs about life and death and different faiths and cultures deal with loss and death in their own distinctive ways. In some communities, death is seen as one step in the continuous cycle of life whereas in others it is seen as an ending. How individuals respond to loss will therefore depend on a multiplicity of factors. It may nonetheless be useful to consider some theories of grief and loss which can be used to inform the support that staff can offer to children, young people and their families.

A number of theories explore and attempt to describe the experiences of grief, loss and bereavement. Whilst these tend to focus on experiences associated with death, the same processes, or theories, can be extended to the adjustment to loss and feelings of grief that occur when a child or young person has complex and continuing health needs.

Amongst the theories related to loss is that of Kübler Ross (1997) who describes the experience of grief in stages which an individual may experience following loss: denial, anger, bargaining, depression and acceptance. This model has served as a useful guide to many individuals and professionals and has assisted people to gain insight into what they feel following loss and why. However, the theory has been debated and often criticised for simplifying the complexity of individual's responses to loss and suggesting a logical and linear progression to acceptance of these. Kübler Ross (1997) herself clarified that the stages are not intended to be seen as concrete, linear, sequential or easily definable. Rather, they intend to give insight into what people may feel when they experience loss, and to enable them and others to understand these feelings.

Other writers suggest that rather than moving through stages, grief requires individuals to accomplish a series of tasks. For example, Worden (1991) describes the tasks of grief as including accepting the reality of loss, experiencing the pain of grief, adjusting to an environment without the person who has died (or, in the case of a child who has complex health needs without the person or aspects of life that were known or expected) and relocating the person who has died or the aspects of life which have been lost emotionally and moving on with life. Whilst this model differs from Kübler Ross's in that it describes tasks, rather than stages, it still tends to describe a linear process, or progression, with a view to final resolution and acceptance of life without a person who has died or an aspect of life which has been lost.

More recent theories have suggested that a grief is more complex than such models suggest, highly individual, and incompletely understood (Krueger 2006). Krueger (2006) places emphasis on the need for a meaning to be made of the loss which has been experienced, and the very individual way in which personal narratives have to be rewritten and values shifted following loss. Where a child or young person has complex health needs, this may include searching for a reason for the child's condition or a diagnosis to try to make meaning and sense of the situation. It may also involve inner searching by parents as they try to identify what this means for them and what their future will be. The expected narrative of their life with their child may require significant revision. They may need to change the value which they place on certain aspects of life, and what is important to them and what will be possible for them in life. Their expected future may need to be reviewed and rewritten, and what life meant for them and their family reviewed (Barr and Millar 2003).

Where a child has died, it is likely that almost every aspect of their parents' life will require reconstruction as their parents would have expected their child to be a part of their entire life (Rosenblatt 2000). This may mean that throughout their lives they come across situations or experiences which they have to revise, and which cause them to recall what they had expected or hoped for. Similarly, where a child has or develops complex health needs, the expected narratives for them and their family may have to be constantly readjusted as they get older, their condition changes or as service provision or facilities for them alter.

If a person dies, Walter (1996) suggests that the bereaved need to construct a meaningful, ongoing biography of them, so that they can integrate their memory into their continuing lives. Rather than moving on, Krueger (2006) suggests that individuals have to learn to love the person who is dead in a different way from the person who was alive. In the case of parents whose child has died, this enables them to hold on to their relationship with their child, rather than letting go and to understand the continuing influence of the child on their lives, rather than trying to develop a life without them (Davies 2004). These approaches differ from the linear model, insofar as they focus on how the person who has died or the situation of loss can be incorporated into the ongoing lives of those affected by their loss, rather than their loss and the emotions associated with this being resolved.

CHILDREN AND YOUNG PEOPLE'S CONCEPTS OF DEATH

As well as being aware of some of the theories related to loss, it may be useful for those who are supporting a child who believes they will die, or their siblings, to have some insight into a child's or young person's concept of death. Each child's understanding of death will vary according to their age, cognitive level, and previous experiences of illness or death (Dyregrov 2002). Living with long-term illness or disability or having a sibling who has a long-term illness or disability is likely to change a child's perceptions and insights related to a range of life events, including health, illness, and death. It often makes them more aware of issues related to these than they would usually be at a given age.

Identifying the understanding a child or young person who has complex health needs has of death is sometimes very difficult. This may be because communication difficulties make it hard to determine their understanding, or because their cognitive level is not thought to be what would be expected at their age. However, even where a child has a cognitive ability which may be less than expected at a given age, their health status may sometimes mean that they still have a greater awareness than might be expected of death. The guidance given on the usual, or likely, understanding of death at any given age may not, therefore, be neatly transferred to children and young people who have complex health needs and their siblings. It may nonetheless provide some insights into the way in which children may understand and respond to death.

Children under the age of five are not thought to understand that death is final. However, they can sense when there is sadness around them and when a significant person is missing, and respond very strongly to loss (Paediatric Intensive Care Society 2002). Even below the age of two children are aware of and can express ideas about people not being there anymore and can think that they caused death or other misfortunes, or that they can reverse this process (Dyregrov 2002). They may see death as a punishment for bad behaviour (for example, siblings may think that their behaviour has caused their sibling's illness or death, and a child who has developed a health problem or believes that they will die may feel that it is a punishment for some wrongdoing) (Paediatric Intensive Care Society 2002).

Between the ages of five and 10 children gradually become aware of the irreversibility of death, and that everyone will one day die. They begin to show compassion for others in relation to loss and begin to become concerned with injustice. For example, at this age children may feel the injustice of their sibling's health needs, the opportunities which they lose, or how people treat them, or their death. At this stage they may also begin to be less willing to share their feelings with other people, especially adults (Dyergrov 2002).

Above the age of 10, a young person's concept of death becomes closer to the adult understanding, and they have a greater awareness of the long-term consequences of loss through death as well as the loss of the person's immediate presence. They begin to reflect more on justice, injustice and fate (Dyergrov 2002). Their developing independence may, at the same time, mean that they are reluctant to share their feelings with others, especially with their family, but it is important that they have the chance to discuss what they are experiencing and feeling.

Children who are faced with loss may cope with or respond to this in a number of ways, depending on a range of factors, including their age and understanding of events related to long-term illness and death, the circumstances of their loss, how other family members respond to the situation, how the family is affected, their own and their family's religious or spiritual and cultural beliefs, and their own feelings of self-worth. Children, especially young children, may not seem not to understand or take in news of loss, or may appear to carry on with life as if this is unimportant. This may be because they do not understand the finality of the loss (Dyergrov 2002). It may also be because they do not know how to respond. Children and young people, like adults, may experience shock and disbelief when confronted with loss, and may not take in everything at once, or know what to do or say. They may also feel unable to cope with the way in which those around them are responding, and may feel guilt because they perceive they may be to blame, and that others will blame them. They may need repeated explanations over time to enable them to understand the information, and what this means, and should have the chance to think about what they have been told, or what has happened, and to ask questions about it and to share their feelings.

Children's capacity to sustain or demonstrate sad emotions increases with age and maturity. An apparent lack of ongoing sadness in children may lead adults to believe they are unaffected by the loss they have experienced, or have recovered from this. However, even when a child does not appear to be sad any more, they often are, and responses to loss may manifest months or even years after the event. Children and young people, like adults, revisit grief at different stages of their development and at especially notable times in their lives, or the lives which would have been their sibling's (Dyergrov 2002).

Case study

Lucy's younger sister, Claire, was born prematurely, has residual respiratory problems, and requires CPAP at night. She also has cerebral palsy. Lucy is five. She had been 'promised' that when she got her new sister her mother would be gone for a day or two, but that she could go with her father and see her new sister, and then her sister would come home and she would be able to help her mother to bath and dress her. However, none of this happened. Instead, she says: 'I had to go and live at Nanny's for a while. I missed Mummy and Daddy, but they were with Claire, not me. I was meant to help them dress her, and bath her, but I was at Nanny's so I couldn't. I think maybe because I didn't really want a sister, I wanted a puppy, I didn't get one. In the end I did want a sister, but at first I wanted a puppy.'

Lucy's mother recalls: 'When I was pregnant with Claire, we had promised Lucy she could help me with her when she was born. Things like bathing her and dressing her. Lucy hadn't really been very keen on a sister at first, but she got really excited about her in the end. Then when Claire was born so early, and was so sick, she couldn't see her really, or touch her, and we were at the hospital and she had to go to my Mum's. Mum said to me "Don't worry, she doesn't mind. She isn't worried about her sister. She just asked: Can we have the puppy now, if the baby isn't coming home?" So, we thought she was OK. Then later on we asked her, because she had had such a hard time, and had been so good, did she want a puppy. She just cried and said: "Don't want a puppy. I want to have the baby."'

Some responses which have been reported in children who have suffered loss include: anxiety, vivid memories (for example of the sibling who has died), difficulty sleeping, fear of going to sleep, nightmares, guilt, self-reproach and longing for the person who has died or the part of their life which is lost. Children may also experience physical ill health, have poor concentration, poor memory, and regress in relation to previously learned skills (Dyergrov 2002; Paediatric Intensive Care Society 2002). They may also demonstrate altered behaviour, for example, being unusually quiet and withdrawn, demanding attention or being clingy, being jealous of other children, being angry, aggressive or having tantrums, finding it difficult to play with other children, or playing in a repetitive way, especially about their loss (Paediatric Intensive Care Society 2002). Children may in some cases appear more 'adult' than expected during or following loss and may try to protect their parents by suppressing their own grief (Paediatric Intensive Care Society 2002). This may lead people to believe that they are coping well, but they still need the opportunity to be supported themselves.

For all children of whatever age, loss and grief are very individual experiences, and the presence of supportive adults to help them explore their feelings is important (Gilroy and Johnson 2004). They may prefer to talk to an adult other than their parents about their feelings, and healthcare professionals may need to explain this to their parents, to help them not to feel rejected by other children at the same time as dealing with their existing losses.

Enabling children or young people who have complex health needs to discuss their own anticipated death, or a friend or peer's death away from their parents may be difficult to organise if their parents provide for all their care needs or assist greatly with all their needs. Where the child or young person has specific communication needs, this may be even more difficult, but remains equally as important as for any other child.

Children may be scared by their reactions to loss, and may need reassurance that these are normal. This includes times when they forget about their loss. They may also need permission to play with friends and do normal things and continued reassurance that they are loved (Paediatric Intensive Care Society 2002). Although it is sometimes suggested that children whose sibling has died should be reassured that they will not die (Paediatric Intensive care Society 2002), this may be less straightforward in the case of children with genetic disorders that their siblings also have or may have. Siblings may, in such cases, have the very realistic fear that they too have or will have this disorder and will also die. In some instances they may know this to be the case. In other cases, siblings may wonder about their own children having the disorder and the impact on their long-term plans and relationships. In such situations it will be expedient for them to be able to discuss their concerns with someone with knowledge of the disease in question, and who has confidence to discuss such matters with children and young people.

FAMILIES LIVING WITH LOSS

When a child dies, or develops a disorder that is likely to shorten their life, their parents have to deal with their personal grief, concern for their other children, and with the needs of the child themselves (deCinque et al. 2006). Equally, children's grief can be confounded by concern for their parents and siblings (Paediatric Intensive Care Society 2002). The whole family has to cope with their emotions, and as every individual copes, manages, or learns to live with, their loss in a different way, and at a different pace, it is likely that these will vary within the family unit (Parkes and Markus 1998). Family members may respond differently to loss, loss may mean different things to them, and they may have different ways of addressing their loss. They may also experience the same feelings or have the same ways of managing their feelings as one another, but at different times and at different paces to each other. This can cause conflict if individuals perceive that other family members are responding inappropriately, inadequately or do not understand their feelings or care about the loss which the family has sustained. This may be a source of conflict or breakdown of understanding within families.

If a member of the family was involved in the incident which caused death or injury, their feelings of guilt about this (for example where a child was involved in a road traffic accident where one of the parents was driving), how the other parent feels about the incident, and the support available to them will influence their ability to come to terms with the situation. This may also apply to genetic defects if only one parent is affected.

Thus, as well as the loss itself, the way in which grief and loss is experienced by individuals within families may impact on family communication, understanding and functioning and may lessen or worsen the stress which the family as a whole experience. Whilst the merits of various models of grief and loss are debated, they may be helpful in assisting families to understand their own responses to loss, their feelings, those of other family members, and the reality that these are likely to vary.

Case study

Sofia and Pietro had two daughters, Alessia and Serena. Alessia had multiple disabilities, and has recently died. Serena is 16. Sofia cared for Alessia, with only occasional assistance. She is now organising her funeral and memorial service, but describes how: 'Every part of the day, I was thinking of Alessia and Serena, looking after Alessia, and Serena too, but she had much less need. She was four when Alessia was born. People think, and some even say to me: "You had a hard life, now that Alessia is gone, it must be easier. You can get your life back. What they don't realise is that she was such a big part of my life; she was my companion as much as I was hers. I miss her every minute. I honestly don't know what I am going to do without her. I spent so much of my day with her, she was such a lovely girl, and I loved her so much.'

Pietro had two days of leave from work after Alessia died, but has now returned, because there is nothing he can do at home. He feels very ambivalent about Alessia's death. He always knew she would die, and that the time of her death was approaching. He feels that he had grieved for her over the years of her life, and her death is not a sudden change, but rather the next stage of his grief. He is also acutely aware that the family may now have a more normal life. At the same time, he is aware that his wife misses their daughter, as he does.

Serena misses her sister a great deal. She used to spend a lot of time with her, helping her mother but also reading to Alessia, and watching TV with her. She was very attached to her, loved her smile and her gentle personality. She explains how: 'She was someone I could always talk to. She couldn't reply, but I could think aloud with her. She knew all my secrets.' However, she always felt that she grew up in Alessia's shadow, and sometimes felt that Alessia, through no fault of her own, meant she could not be like her friends. She feels guilty that a small part of her knows she no longer has to worry about her future with Alessia.

SUPPORTING FAMILIES WHO EXPERIENCE LOSS

Whilst providing support in relation to loss is a part of the role that healthcare staff may have in supporting children, young people and their families, it is also important to recognise that families may have their own social support networks which exclude healthcare professionals. The time at which families most need support varies, some may never want support from outsiders, and the time at which families want support may not always be in the immediate time following the child's death or the discovery of a life-limiting illness. For example, when a child is diagnosed as having a long-term life-limiting illness their parents may not, after the diagnosis is given, initially wish to access support from healthcare staff, support groups or other professional services. They may prefer to deal with the issues involved and their feelings within the family group or with the support of close friends. However, at a later stage, they may wish to access more information and support from individual professionals or support groups. Refusal of input should not, therefore, be seen as a permanent event and channels of communication should be left open for support at a later stage. The role of healthcare professionals is to provide whatever assistance the family requires, in a flexible manner, and to ensure that they are aware of how ongoing support can be accessed (Paediatric Intensive Care Society 2002).

The need to balance intrusion with support in every aspect of supporting families applies equally, if not more, to times when they are experiencing loss. Given the number of things that may create feelings of loss for children and young people who have complex health needs and their families, this may be an almost constant state of being for some. This emphasises the need for staff to be constantly sensitive to the necessity of being supportive, available, but not intrusive.

Providing an opportunity for families where a child has died to talk about them is a very important part of supporting them. Assisting and enabling parents to explore the significance of their child's life, and their continuing influence on their own lives may assist them in making sense of their loss and rewriting the narrative of their own and their family's life (Davies 2004). It is often difficult for families to find people who are willing to talk with them in this way, and some families do not find it easy to talk to people who do not have the same experience as them. The provision of details of support groups who may be able to provide this type of peer understanding may be invaluable for families (Davies 2004).

Support groups that relate to the child or young person's needs can be very important for families, but when a child dies, at a time when the family need support from peers, they may feel disqualified from using such groups. They may also be aware of the likely impact of their loss on other group members which may disincline them from continuing to participate or may feel that because their child is no longer alive they are not entitled to continue to participate. Other support mechanisms may also be lost at a time when they could benefit from these, such as support from other parents at the child's school, school staff, and the range of health and social care staff who were involved with the family while the child was alive. How ongoing support may be provided is therefore something that should be considered if a child or young person is expected to die or dies following long-term illness, and directing parents to support groups where they can discuss their child's life and death, and their implications, may again be very useful.

One fundamental principle when a child is expected to die is to tell the truth (Paediatric Intensive Care Society 2002). The same applies when information about a poor prognosis, or disability is given. However, this must be done in a manner that is supportive and likely to minimise distress for the family concerned. What happens at the time of the child's death or the discussion of diagnosis and prognosis can have lifelong repercussions and many families recall very clearly being given information on their child's disability and prognosis in a cold, callous or uncaring way. Equally, when this is done sensitively, families recall and often find great comfort in it (Hewitt-Taylor 2007). In the case of children who have complex and continuing health needs, the way in which information is given may affect how well their parents are able to adjust to the child's illness and cope with the demands that their care makes on them. It may also affect all their relationships with healthcare workers and their inclination to trust healthcare staff and seek ongoing help and support from them.

Parents whose children have complex health needs may require assistance and support regarding the practicalities associated with their child's death

(Department of Health 2004a). Whilst, as discussed in Chapter 3, having a child who has complex health needs can cause financial problems for families, their child dying may create further financial difficulties for them. If they have been their child's main carer, they lose the financial allowances and state benefits which they received for this. At the same time, they have to meet funeral expenses and other costs related to their child's death. This often follows a period of time when the family has already struggled financially because of the cost of their child's needs (Corden et al. 2002). Parents who have been unable to work may find that re-engaging with employment can be a slow and difficult process for them. Although they may have had a well-paid job prior to taking on the responsibility for caring for their child, they are unlikely to be able to swiftly or easily regain employment, especially at the same level at which they left. Resuming employment will often be difficult because of their time out of the workplace, but also because they will be grieving for their child at the same time as seeking work (Corden et al. 2002).

Healthcare staff may be able to assist in pointing parents in the right direction for financial advice and support and where a child is not expected to live it may be appropriate to include such considerations in preparing parents for the child's inevitable death. It also emphasises the importance of support being organised to enable parents to continue in employment whilst caring for their child if they wish to do so.

LOSS FOR HEALTHCARE STAFF

Working closely with a child and family in their home over a long period of time is, as identified in chapters four and five, a very different experience to many other types of care work. It can mean that staff and families become much closer and share a great deal more of their lives and experiences than they do in other situations (Samwell 2005). Staff may feel much closer to the child and family, and may feel the losses that a child, young person or their family experience acutely, for example, when they reach a new stage of illness, lose an opportunity, are discriminated against, or die.

Staff who support parents whose children have complex health needs may themselves be grieving for the child or young person and their family's losses as well as trying to support them. It is important that they too have recourse to support in such circumstances (Serwint 2004; Bartlow 2006). Although staff who work closely with families need to achieve the delicate balance between concern and over-involvement, they also need to acknowledge their own humanity and needs when they experience loss related to their work.

Case study

Chandra worked with Zena and her family for ten years. She got on very well with them and recalls how: "One day, we went shopping with Zena, I heard some teengaers laughing at her, and I wanted to go and tell them off, but Hilary (Zena's Mum) said 'No, leave them. Let's just enjoy ourselves. Don't let them spoil our day.' She was right, but I felt so hurt for Zena and so angry that they would behave like that. Then when she wasn't offered a place at college, I felt really upset, because I thought she deserved that chance. I knew how well she could have done. I worked with her for ten years. Then she died, of a chest infection, just after she should have started college, if she'd had the chance. It was like a big part of my life was gone. I really felt I lost a friend. Not just Zena, but the family too, because you don't like to just keep calling in, because I was only there for Zena, and it seems a bit odd to stick around. They have their lives, and so do I, but I do feel like a part of me, and my life, has gone."

SUMMARY

Children and young people who have complex health needs and their families may experience loss and grief because of a variety of life events, both related to their health needs and unrelated to these. Staff who work with children, young people and their families should be alert to the huge range of issues which may cause or contribute to them experiencing loss or feelings of grief. At the same time, assumptions should not be made about what may or may not cause feelings of loss, and how people may respond to these, as these are highly individual.

As well as supporting children and their families, and facilitating them accessing specialist support, staff should be aware that they too may need an opportunity to discuss their feelings and gain support related to the losses that a child or young person and their family experience, or which they experience in relation to their work.

Chapter 8
Choices and Rights

In order to provide support that focuses on the needs, wishes and priorities of children, young people and their families those who work with them need to appreciate the rights that they have. This includes clarity over the right a child or young person has to make informed choices about their life, and for their decisions to be respected and acted on. At the same time, staff need to be aware of their responsibilities, for example in cases where there is a difference between the child or young person's views and those of their parents and professionals.

This chapter discusses some of the rights which children, young people, and their families have, how these apply to children and young people who have complex and continuing health needs, and how they should influence the support that they receive.

CHILDREN'S RIGHTS

Until the late twentieth century children were largely seen as their parents' property, with few rights of their own (Rowse 2007). However, children's rights have now been recognised in a number of documents, and the child's best interests are seen as being of paramount importance in all the decisions in which they are concerned (Office of the United Nations High Commissioner for Human Rights 1989; Department of Health 2004b).

The United Nations Convention on the Rights of the Child is intended to give children worldwide an equal right to certain standards of life and safety (Rowse 2007). This convention has been ratified by the UK Government, which allows it to be used as an argument in English Law (Rowse 2007). It is not directly enforceable in courts, but its ratification means that the UK Government has agreed to do everything possible to implement it, and that observance of the convention's principles is monitored (Dimond 2005). The Children Act (Department of Health 2004b) also provides a legal basis for the enforcement of some parts of the convention.

The European Convention on Human Rights was enacted to protect fundamental human rights and freedoms. The tenets of this convention are incorporated in The Human Rights Act (HMSO 1998), which came into force in the United Kingdom in 2000. This means that the European Convention on Human Rights is directly enforceable in courts in England and Wales (Dimond 2005). In addition, British Citizens can seek protection through the European Court of Human Rights in Strasbourg. The rights that all citizens have through the Human Rights Act apply equally to children and young people who have complex health needs.

The United Nations Convention on the Rights of the Child (Article 12) and the Children Act (Department of Health 2004b) afford children and young people who are capable of forming their own views the right to express these freely in all matters affecting them. They also give children and young people the right to have these views heard and given due weight, in accordance with their age and maturity. Whilst this provides clear recognition of the child or young person's right to be involved in decisions about them, it also means that whether they are capable of making their own decisions, what the due weight which their views should be given is, and how these are to be determined must be decided. In essence, this concerns how and by whom the child's degree of autonomy is to be determined.

AUTONOMY

Autonomy can be defined as an individual's ability to make self-determining choices. It involves them being independent, having the capacity to reason, and being able to make decisions (Lowden 2002). A person who has diminished autonomy is in some respect incapable of making decisions or acting on their decisions, and is subject to some degree of control by others (Moser et al. 2007). However, there are a variety of ways in which an individual's autonomy may be decreased. It may be useful to distinguish personal autonomy, which is concerned with the capacity for self-governance or the ability to make decisions and choices, and actual self-governance or the ability to carry out one's choices or decisions. A person may be able to cognitively weigh up the various aspects of a situation and make a decision, but be unable to act on their decision unless others are prepared to assist them to make their choices a reality. This may relate to small, everyday choices, or major life decisions.

Case study

Maria is 17. She has very limited mobility, and requires assisted ventilation. She lives at home, with her mother, Naomi, and her 10-year-old sister Anita. The family are provided with carers overnight and while Maria is at college. Maria also has three weekends a year short-break care. Maria recently decided that she would like to learn to play chess, and join the college chess club which meets after college on Mondays. However, her carers finish work at 4 pm, and her transport home is arranged for straight after college. Unless someone can escort her and her transport can be rearranged, she will not be able to act on her decision to learn to play alongside her peers. She explains: 'Of course I can teach myself, get a swanky computer to play on, but I find I learn things better alongside other people, so I would have preferred to do it that way.'

The concept of autonomy in terms of a child or young person's right to make decisions related to their healthcare and to have these acted on can be very complex. It needs to take into account not only the child or young person's right to make decisions, but the rights which parents and other adults have in relation to them (Bridges et al. 2001; Edgar et al. 2001). Parental rights, as described in Chapter 3, mean the rights, duties, power, responsibilities and authority which, by law, a child's parent has related to the child and their property (Department of Health 2004b). A parent does not have rights over their child, because a child is an individual in their own right, not the property of another person. However, those with parental responsibility do have the right to make decisions about and on behalf of their child (Cormack 2007). These rights include the right to give consent to medical treatment on behalf of their child and to make decisions about their healthcare. However, children and young people also have the right to make their own decisions about healthcare in some circumstances. One of the complexities of discussions on the rights of children and young people in decision making about healthcare is that it is sometimes necessary to decide whether the child or young person, or their parents, has the greatest right to request, consent or refuse treatment or care.

When there is an apparent difference of opinion between children or young people, their parents and healthcare staff over the care, interventions or treatment that they should receive, perhaps the first and most important point is to identify the reasons for each person's views. Differences in opinion may be because of differing perspectives on quality of life, and what will contribute to this. For example, parents' wishes to sustain their child's life may be driven by a desire to have more time with them, even though they know that their child will die before them. Medical staff may see a severely disabled child, who has a very limited life expectancy and physical abilities, but the child's parents may see a child who loves music and responds positively to touch and being in water, who still enjoys these qualities of life, and with whom they enjoy being (Rowse 2007). Healthcare staff may see the formation of a gastrostomy as the best way to ensure the child's physical well-being, but parents may see this as giving in (Hazel 2006) and it may mean the cessation of the enjoyment that they and their child derive from eating and the social events around this (Hewitt-Taylor 2007). Children, young people, their parents and healthcare staff may all have differing views on what constitutes quality of life, and what will contribute to this and thus on different perspectives on the relative merits of aspects of treatment, interventions and care.

Although the child's well-being is paramount, what is deemed to be well-being is debatable. As Chapters 2 and 3 have discussed, well-being means different things to different people. A child or their parent failing to consent to what healthcare staff believe to be the child's best physical health option may not be equivalent to them opting for a course of action that is not in the child or young person's best interests. They may be opting for a different type of well-being which is more important to them. It could be seen as being against the child or young person's best interests and detrimental to their well-being to coerce or insist on them having treatment or care which they and their parents do not wish to consent to or which will lead to an outcome they do not value or which is not their priority.

When a difference of opinion exists concerning whether interventions, care, or support should be provided it is therefore important to ascertain what values, beliefs and priorities each person has, how they have weighed these up, and what matters to them. In addition, if treatment, care or interventions appear to be refused it is important to ascertain what a child or young person is refusing and why. For example, whether their reluctance is about a procedure or an outcome: a child may express disinclination to a painful procedure, but may want the outcome in terms of freedom from pain, improved health, mobility, or quality of life. In contrast, their main concern may not be the short-term discomfort of an intervention, but concerns over the long term implications of this.

Case study

Natasha is eight years old. She has required assisted ventilation at night for some years, but has recently been getting more chest infections, which are increasingly difficult to resolve. At present her assisted ventilation is provided via a nasal mask. Clearing her secretions seems to be a problem, and she has a fairly weak cough. The medical team have suggested that a tracheostomy might be beneficial for her, as they are not sure how effective the seal she achieves on her nasal mask is, and a tracheostomy would possibly facilitate more effective respiratory support and better removal of secretions.

Natasha's mother, Faye, is reluctant for Natasha to have a tracheostomy performed. Natasha is very sociable, and her speech might be affected by having a tracheostomy (they have been told that Natasha would need to learn to use a speaking tube, and that there is a chance that she would be unable to speak). She also realises that there would be some activities which Natasha enjoys, such as swimming, which would not be available to her if she had a tracheostomy. She wants the best for Natasha, and is very worried about her current chest problems. However, she does not want to make a decision that stops Natasha enjoying parts of her life which are important to her, especially as the outcome of having the tracheostomy is uncertain, and the benefit not definite. Although Natasha has had a number of chest infections, Faye is not convinced that this is not just 'bad luck' and linked to the fact that Natasha's brother, Adam, who is three, has just started pre-school and is 'bringing every bug imaginable home with him'.

Natasha does not want to have a tracheostomy. She is reluctant to undergo surgery and prolonged hospitalisation, is very concerned that her tracheostomy, unlike her nasal mask, will be there 'all day as well as all night' and that she may be unable to speak. She also knows that it means she will need to have suction, and to take extra equipment with her wherever she goes. She will be more 'different' than she is now and more restricted in her activities.

Ultimately, the debate on whose view holds the most weight, or will be acted on, related to healthcare becomes an issue of a child or young person's ability to consent or withold consent for healthcare interventions. This requires consideration of their autonomy in relation to decision making in healthcare.

AUTONOMY AND HEALTHCARE

Respecting individuals' autonomy has become a major theme in healthcare (Joffe et al. 2003; Sullivan 2003). This is a significant change from the stance which has historically permeated healthcare provision, in which healthcare staff, and in particular medical staff, made decisions on behalf of patients (Kennedy 2003).

Gallant et al. (2002) suggest that the change from medical staff making decisions on behalf of others to a focus on the autonomy of health service users has occurred because of an increase in democratic thinking in healthcare, and seeking to honour basic human rights in healthcare relationships. However, greater respect for the autonomy of those using health services may also have become a necessity in a society in which deference is no longer unquestioningly given to medical staff (Wilmot 2003). Kennedy (2003) identifies that in British culture individuals are now more aware of their rights, expect to be given information, and to make their own decisions about every aspect of their lives. This has been accompanied by a loss of confidence in medicine following well-publicised cases of misconduct (Canter 2001), the challenging of the biomedical model of health (Wilmot 2003) and cases where expertise has been found to be wanting, or decisions made by healthcare staff overturned in favour of parents' views (Dyer 2004). Although a move towards greater respect for autonomy in healthcare is often described, whether this is true respect for the autonomy of service users, or the public declining to accommodate medical paternalism, and policy and practice being required to shift in acknowledgment of this is debatable.

Respect for autonomy should be a fundamental part of the relationship between healthcare staff and service users. However, this should not be equated with health service providers being unconcerned for service users or an abdication of responsibility for providing them with information and support. Orfali and Gordon (2004) report how the emphasis on respect for parental autonomy on an American neonatal unit appeared to create limited rapport between medical staff and parents to the extent of parents feeling isolated and unsupported in making very difficult decisions about their babies. This lack of what has been described as 'emotional work' in promoting autonomy indicates a need for the right to autonomy to be a part of trusting, caring relationships, in which open and honest but supportive information giving happens, and children, young people and their families are supported in finding the best decision for them.

Although autonomy is concerned with self-determination, a person who acts autonomously can seek and accept advice, support and assistance from others, and can also choose to defer to others. The key in autonomous decision making is that an individual has the right to make their own decisions, and to decide how much influence others have in their decision making (Kaplan 2002; Lowden 2002). This may include seeking information from others, asking others their views and opinions, and even allowing others to make decisions for them. However, the influence afforded to the views of others, and their involvement in the decision-making process is the individual's choice, not imposed on them.

Case study

Faye describes how she feels about the decision making that she and her daughter are engaged in: 'It's like, it is our choice, but they think they are right. I can see that they think that, and maybe medically they are, but no one really listens to our concerns. They just repeat what they have already said about her breathing. What

I want is for someone to sit down with us and discuss this, to let me say what my concerns are and why, so that they understand and can talk to me about those. I'm not just wanting to avoid her having a trache because it's more work, or she can't swim, it's about her whole quality of life and how she feels. Whatever we decide, I want to really be sure I did the right thing. Right now I feel as if yes, they do say it's our choice, but I feel as if, if I say no, and she ends up in ICU again, they will say "We told you so." I do take responsibility for my decisions, but I feel as if I will be really a persona non gratis if we call the wrong shot and she gets sick again. But I don't want to make the wrong choice, just because I'm afraid of being in disgrace with the doctors. I know they feel I have got Natasha to worry about it, but it's really the other way round. The things I ask about are what she is worried about too. If she was happy to go ahead, I would be. She was the one who asked me about swimming. I didn't suggest it.'

COMPETENCE IN DECISION MAKING

A major issue in determining the weight that will be given to children and young people's views related to their health is whether or not they are deemed to be competent. As identified previously, those with parental responsibility for a child have the right to make certain decisions on their behalf, but in some circumstances children and young people have the right to make their own decisions. The mainstay of whether and to what extent they have this right is their competence to make the decision or decisions in question.

Competence relates to the ability to perform specific tasks, and children and young people may therefore be deemed to be competent in some respects, or in some situations, but not in others. To be competent to consent to treatment or other aspects of healthcare, a child or young person must be able to make the decision related to the particular intervention, treatment or care in question (Edwards 1996). An individual may be able to reason and to make decisions, but in order to make decisions regarding their health, they need sufficient information (Christensen and Hewitt-Taylor 2006). This means them having information they can understand regarding the interventions, treatment or care in question, including the likely outcomes, any alternative options, and the implications of not receiving the treatment or care. It also necessitates children and young people being given the opportunity to ask questions and discuss the options involved so as to determine what they believe will be best for them (Lowden 2002).

Simply providing information does not guarantee that the recipient has understood this, or that the information is unbiased (Mandana 2007). If information is conveyed in terms that are overly complex or unfamiliar, the child or young person concerned's ability to achieve competence will be impaired. If adults are unwilling to listen, or are unable to understand the child or young person's way of expressing themselves, their views may be disregarded even when they want to make their own decisions and are competent to consent (Lowden 2002). Those working with children, young people, and their families have a responsibility to convey information in a manner that is appropriate for the child's age, developmental level, and understanding of the issue in question. Where a child has altered communication, the information must be delivered in a way that they will be able to access. Those who work with them must be able and willing to listen and to create the opportunity for them to communicate, not only to convey their choices, but to discuss the information that has been presented to them (Lowden 2002). This may be challenging in any child, and may be particularly so where a child or young person cannot communicate verbally. However, the challenges that it presents are not a reason to disregard a child or young person's rights, and differences in the ways in which people communicate should not be equated with a decreased ability to make decisions.

Whilst information giving is an essential part of enabling individuals to achieve autonomy in decision making, Canter (2001) identifies that it is not easy to give information without any influence from one's own interpretation of this and beliefs regarding it. However, healthcare professionals should acknowledge that they do not have a completely unbiased view of the evidence, or possess complete and irrefutable knowledge, and should be prepared to enter into discussions in which uncertainties and conflicting views can be explored. Where uncertainty exists, and clear-cut answers cannot be given, this should be made clear, and different viewpoints explored rather than a certainty which does not exist being suggested (Hewitt-Taylor 2007).

Case study

Faye describes how: 'When they said: "Well, maybe it's come to the time when we need to think about doing a trache." Natasha sat and listened to them, about how she had been getting so many infections, how she didn't seem to get on so well with her mask. Then it was her that asked "A tracheostomy . . . that's a hole in your neck. So, what would happen when I go swimming? Is there something like a plug you can put in it?" She was the one asking the questions. She asked: "How do I talk with a trache?" She has seen other people with traches and having suction, so she asked about that. I asked a few things too, but Natasha understands this. Even though she's only eight, and she is quite small, she understands things like this. Last time we saw the consultant she asked him: "Why is there a hurry to decide? I think I could just try the mask a bit longer and see how I go." That was what I was thinking, but she said it. It was her idea.'

CONSENT

Whether or not a child or young person is competent to make a decision is the mainstay of the weight which is given to their views. Children's ability to consent to treatment, interventions or care is dependent on their competence, as decribed in the previous section. However, their legal rights in this respect are not entirely clear. The Children Act (Department of Health 2004b) identifies that children should always be consulted (subject to their age and understanding) and kept informed about what will happen to them. However, in legal terms, there is no real clarity over when a child or young person can consent, or perhaps more importantly withold consent, to treatment, care, or interventions. The Family Law Reform Act 1969 states that a child of 16 or 17 years of age has a statutory right to give consent to medical, surgical and dental treatment. However, a parent can also give consent on behalf of a child up to the age of 18 and if a child aged 16 or 17 refuses treatment that is deemed by others to be in their best interests, their refusal can be overruled by their parents or by the courts (Dimond 2005).

When children under the age of 16 are involved in decision making about medical treatment their legal rights are governed by common law (Parekh 2006). Below the age of 16, a child does not have the statutory right to give consent to treatment, but the House of Lords has held that if a child is competent to understand the nature of the proposed treatment and its effects then they can give valid consent to treatment (*Gillick* vs *West Norfolk and Wisbech Health Authority 1986*). This has become termed 'Gillick competence'. A Gillick competent child is one who is deemed to have the capacity to give informed consent, having received the relevant information, understood and balanced it and made the decision that this is what they want. The age at which a child becomes Gillick competent therefore depends on their understanding of the treatment in question and its likely consequences (Parekh 2006).

Whilst a child under the age of 16 can consent to treatment, if they refuse treatment, until they are 18 their parents may consent on their behalf, or the courts may overturn their and their parents' refusal if it is deemed to be in the child's best interests to do so (Parekh 2006). Thus, a child or young person under the age of 18 can never refuse teatment without questioning. This means that no child is allowed to be fully autonomous in decision making about their health, as they can consent to, but not decline, treatment (Lowden 2002; Parekh 2006). This leaves in question why a child could be competent to consent to, but not to refuse treatment. It also brings into question the value of allowing a child to consent to treatment when, unless their right to consent includes the right to refuse treatment, consent is no more than the right to agree with medical practitioners or their parents.

Determining when a child or young person is competent to consent can be complex, and where lack of clarity exists over a child or young person's rights in this respect legal advice may be sought. However, Parekh (2006) suggests that the way in which children's competence is assessed should involve a more holistic approach than only medical and legal staff being involved in the decision. Instead, those who know them best, possibly including nurses, sociologists, psychologists, religious or cultural leaders and others should be consulted. The aim should be to gain as in depth as possible an idea of the child or young person's understanding of the situation, their priorities, values and the view that they have of health and well-being. This may be especially important for children and young people who have complex health needs. Their families and those who have worked closely with them or who are familiar with their ways of communicating and are likely to have the greatest awareness of their level of understanding and ability to achieve competence in decision making over any given matter.

Where decisions involve life, death, and the potential for suffering, parents may need to be helped and encouraged to allow their children to be involved in decision making (Lowden 2002). As discussed in Chapter 6, it may be very difficult for parents whose children have complex health needs to accept their independence in healthcare decision making. They may need support in this process, especially if the young person decides on a course of action that seems at odds with the goals which their parents have pursued over many years.

Given the many factors that contribute to competence to consent, how this competence is almost immediately achieved at the age of 18 is questionable (Parekh 2006). Although age is often linked with the right to consent to treatment, experience of relevant treatment or health-related matters has been found to be more important than age in whether or not a child is really competent to consent or withold consent to treatment, care or interventions (Parekh 2006). Children who have complex and continuing health needs, and who have considerable experience of healthcare and interventions, may be much more competent to make decisions about healthcare than 18 year olds who have very limited exposure to personal health related decision making. Even when they have delayed congnitive development, their experiences may mean that children and young people who have complex health needs have a better understanding of health related matters than their peers.

Case study

Omar is 10. He is unable to move unaided, and requires assistance with all his daily care needs. He has hearing problems but can lip-read, and uses symbols, pictures and a switch to communicate. His parents and carers are adept at using these with him.

Omar recently attended an outpatients clinic and the consultant spoke to his mother, Juliana, and stated, amongst other things, that Omar needed some blood taken. He then stood up as if to end the meeting. Juliana's moved to sit opposite Omar, so that he could lip-read her, to explain what the consultant had said, and why he thought that Omar needed blood taken. Omar used his switch to indicate that he understood and that he agreed to have blood taken. Juliana recalls: 'I think he (the consultant) wondered what I was doing. He didn't object, but I think he wondered what was going on. He thought we were about to leave. But Omar understands what is going on, he understands all about his condition, and he should be allowed to say whetehr he wants blood taken, or if he has any questions. He has to send his messages through me a lot of the time, but he can understand, so he should be allowed to ask. Actually, the consultant was very good. He sat down again and said "OK? Is there anything he wants to ask?" I said "No, he says that's fine" then we went, and had the blood taken.'

EMPOWERMENT

Although individuals have the right to autonomy in decision making, they may be unused to being enabled to enjoy this right, and not everyone will embrace their rights in this respect. Children and young people who have complex health needs may therefore need assistance to gain their rights, and to be empowered to act in an autonomous manner. Empowerment has been defined as: 'to give power to, or to make able' (Soanes and Stevenson, 2005). Empowerment occurs when the less powerful are given a chance to gain power and control over specific life experiences (Nyatanga and Dann 2002).

As with the move to promote the autonomy of individuals in healthcare settings, the current aim to empower individuals is a move from the traditional paternalistic stance adopted by medicine. Paternalism can be defined as 'the policy of restricting the freedom and responsibility of subordinates or dependents, in their supposed best interests' (Soanes et al. 2001). In the past, paternalism was the accepted model of medical decision making, and it was often considered inappropriate to burden patients with the onus of decision making regarding their health (Kennedy 2003).

Hewitt (2002) suggests that this view was allowed to persist and was considered justified because the tradition of paternalism meant that it was accepted, and people disinclined to question the way in which medical staff made decisions, or to expect to be involved in decision making about their health. This perpetuated the view that the public were unable to make or be involved in such decisions, and effectively disempowered individuals in healthcare settings.

The trend in medicine is now, at least in theory, away from paternalism, towards a culture of power sharing and respect for individual autonomy (Coulter 1999; Department of Health 2000a). However, although empowering users of healthcare services, like promoting autonomy, is currently a very popular ideal in healthcare, power is not something that can be easily moved from one group or one individual to another (Canter 2001). It is also unlikely that any individual or group with significant power will be easily convinced to yield this to another (Freire 1970). Thus, it is unrealistic to expect that empowerment will be easy to enact. Goodyear-Smith and Buetow (2001) and Tweedale (2003) identify that when service users and medical staff do not agree over the best course of action, paternalism is likely to surface and healthcare staff to try to encourage service users to subscribe to their viewpoint. This echoes the position on children's consent to treatment, insofar as they are permitted to consent whilst they agree with healthcare staff, but their ability to be self-determining is less welcome when their views differ from those of healthcare professionals.

Case study

Faye describes how she feels about the way that medical staff talk to her: 'On the one hand, it's my choice, but when I say what Natasha and I think, what we want, what our concerns are, it's like ... they are cross that we don't agree with them. Maybe not cross, but they think we are wrong and that they know best. They don't explain any more, or listen to me. They don't say it outright but it's like: "Well, it's your choice, but we know best, so if you want what's best for your child, you should really agree with us, because we know what's best."'

It has often been suggested that medical staff are more likely than nurses to act in a disempowering way, with their aim to achieve cure contrasting with nursing's aim for care. However, Salvage (1990) argues that the caring function of nurses can be an equally disempowering force. Their emphasis on care means that nurses may exhibit maternalistic rather than empowering behaviour. Malin and Teasdale (1991) believe that nurses view caring as doing things for people, including protecting them from harm or worry. This, like paternalism, sees the person who requires healthcare as a 'patient' and as unequal to the burden of decision making and taking responsibility for themselves. Hewison (1995) suggests that despite their differences in values and roles, nurses may be no more likely than medical staff to empower patients. They may simply disempower them in a different, and in some respects more subtle and difficult to change way.

Case study

At their last appointment, the consultant suggested to Juliana that they consider Omar having a gastrostomy as oral feeding is becoming increasingly problematic. Juliana has been looking up information on this, and asked one of the nurses who has input into Omar's support to go through it with her and discuss the options. The nurse agreed. When Juliana produced the articles which she had collected and read, and the questions she had, the nurse said: 'Oh, you shouldn't have gone to all that trouble, I know all about this, I can tell you what you need to know. You have enough on!' She then explained what a gastrostomy was, the benefits of a gastrostomy, and how this would help Omar. However, as Juliana explained: 'I wasn't asking her because I didn't understand what I had been told, I was asking her to go through extra information that I had got, to discuss it, all the different views and how they relate to Omar's situation. Really to be a sounding board. I didn't get that. I just got an explanation of what the doctor had already said, but in simple terms. As if I was stupid. This is a really important decision for us, so I don't want soemone else to do my research. I just want someone to bounce ideas around with. I know she meant well, but that was kind of insulting, really.'

ADVOCACY

Although enabling individuals to make autonomous decisions is the aim, some children, young people and their families may be unused to making choices or being involved in decision making, particularly in relation to their healthcare. They may be used to deferring to others, or not being invited or allowed to make choices. For some individuals, the idea of making decisions may be new and threatening, or they may want to be involved in making choices, but require support as they become used to this role. This may be especially so when a child or young person has difficulty in communicating, is not used to being listened to or valued, or feels intimidated by those in authority. It may also be difficult for children, young people and their parents to act autonomously if other people regard them as unable to make autonomous choices.

Children who have complex health needs form a part of what might be described as a vulnerable population: individuals or groups who cannot fully represent and protect their own rights, needs, benefits and wishes, or are unable to carry out their decisions. The way that health professionals sometimes relate to people, for example by disregarding their views or attempts at communicating, or showing disregard for them as people, can further disincline them to attempt to express their views (Mitchell and Bournes 2000). Many children and young people with complex health needs and their families will have had this type of experience.

Whilst it is useful to consider how a person's vulnerability may impair their ability to express autonomous choices, it is also important to ensure that their rights are not violated because of the label 'vulnerable' being applied to them. This type of labelling may mean that they become stigmatised or subject to greater risk of discrimination. It may also predispose to them being treated in the maternalistic, but nonetheless disempowering, way described previously. It is not a person who is vulnerable but rather some aspect of their circumstances that makes them vulnerable at a particular time and in a particular way (McLelland 2006). Thus a person's vulnerability should not be seen as an excuse for paternalistic or maternalistic behaviour, but rather an acknowledgment that they may require specific support to enable them to act autonomously.

Where individuals have difficulty or lack experience or confidence in expressing their wishes or views, or where their voices are likely to remain unheard, an advocate may be useful for them. An advocate may enable an individual who is cognitively able to make their own decisions to achieve this and to have their wishes acted on where it would otherwise be difficult. Advocacy can be defined as 'pleading the cause of another' (Soanes et al. 2001). The National Autistic Society (2007) identify that there are many forms of advocacy, which include: speaking for oneself but with the support of another person, and an individual working one-to-one with another individual and speaking for them by representing the person's interests as if they were the advocate's own. In some situations or organisations, individuals are employed specifically to act in an advocacy role, for example, in legal and healthcare services (Mallik 1998; Grace 2001; MacDonald 2007).

McGrath et al. (2006) consider that advocacy is a core part of nurses' work. However, advocacy exists at many levels and includes: nurses respecting and promoting service users' self-determination; preserving service users' values, benefits, rights, and best interests when they are unable to do this themselves (for example, because they are unconscious); and championing social justice in the provision of healthcare at a wider level by actively striving to achieve changes on behalf of individuals, communities and society (Bu and Jezewski 2006).

Whilst there is a great deal of discussion about of the role of nurses as advocates, there are also some factors which may make this problematic. To be an advocate means that one must be emotionally engaged in the experiences of the person for whom one advocates in order to understand their meaning and thus represent them. This level of understanding of and engagement with a person is crucial in order to assist them to explore and to clarify how they see their situation, determine the decisions that they wish to make, and to present and defend these with them or on their behalf (Gadow 1989). However, it may also be in conflict with nurses' traditional need to maintain some distance from their clients, and to keep the boundaries between them and those with whom they work clear, as discussed in Chapter 4.

Hewitt (2002) also identifies that it is often difficult for nurses to truly distance themselves from their personal or professional beliefs and values, and to advocate for those with whom they work. They may find that loyalties to professional standards, beliefs, values, and the values and beliefs of those with whom they work makes it difficult for them to truly advocate for the children, young people and families with whom they work. Acting as an advocate can also have negative repercussions for individuals if it means them enabling service users to challenge or make decisions that contrast with those of their colleagues (Bu and Jezewski 2006). It may therefore be very difficult for nurses to be truly independent advocates for those with whom they work whilst also maintaining their nursing role. In addition, nurses must consider whether advocating for one person will in any way compromise not only their health, but that of others (Grace 2001). Advocacy in nursing is based on a broader understanding of responsibility and accountability than the one person with whom the nurse is working at any given time, and may therefore make advocating for one child or young person difficult to achieve alongside a nursing role that requires staff to take into account the needs of a wider group of service users and the wider population.

Where children or young people are reliant on staff, they may feel unable to truly express their views or wishes if they feel these are in conflict with those of the staff involved. Thus, although the role of nurses supporting children and their families includes advocacy, it is also necessary for nurses to be aware of when the role of advocate would be better fulfilled by a professional or independent advocate who can devote the whole of their role to advocating for the person, without actual or potential conflicts of interest or role. Like all areas of practice, advocacy, whilst being a core duty of nurses, must be enacted within each individual's personal and professional skills and knowledge. At any point where an individual can no longer fulfil this role to the requisite extent, they should refer to an individual or profession with greater knowledge, skills, expertise, or time and opportunities to fulfil the role.

Case study

Sam is 16. He has required assisted ventilation via a tracheostomy since he was five. He has carers to support him every night, and whilst he is at school, but his family manage the rest of his care. Sam's care package is being reviewed as he approaches the transition to adult services and his family very much want to continue to provide for a great deal of his needs. His carers generally feel that this is very good, and that whilst more support could be made available, if this is the family's choice, this is acceptable, and even laudable, and the best option for Sam. Sam appears to agree with this.

One of Sam's carers has nonetheless suggested that perhaps Sam should have the opportunity to speak through an advocate, because his family may not be representing his views. They care for him very much, and to a very high standard, but she wonders whether, as a young adult, he would prefer greater independence and privacy from his family. It would be difficult for him to express this view as his carers and family are very close to him and often speak for him, and he would not want to hurt his family's feelings by suggesting that he wants to have more independence. She feels that an advocate might enable this to be discussed more effectively.

CHILD PROTECTION

Whilst a great deal of this chapter has been devoted to discussing children's rights in relation to making choices and being afforded autonomy, children also have a right to protection from harm. The welfare of children is always paramount and this principle is upheld in both National Legislation such as the Children Act (Department of Health 2004b), and the United Nations Convention on the Rights of the Child (Office of the United Nations High Commissioner for Human Rights 1989). Article 19 in the United Nations Convention on the Rights of the Child states that:

> States Parties shall take all appropriate legislative, administrative, social and educational measures to protect the child from all forms of physical or mental violence, injury or abuse, neglect or negligent treatment, maltreatment or exploitation, including sexual abuse, while in the care of parent(s), legal guardian(s) or any other person who has the care of the child.

It is a criminal offence to harm a child. Those working with children always have a responsibility to report to the appropriate parties any suspected abuse of children, and clear mechanisms should exist within every organisation concerned about the care of children for this to be achieved.

Although it is always necessary to protect children from harm, one difficulty for staff who work in the family home is determining what is harmful. How individual families conceptualise childhood affects what they see as acceptable childcare practices and what they expect of children in the family (Kelly and Uddin 2005). For example, in some cultures it is expected that siblings will care for their younger brothers or sisters, or have a significant role in their care, whilst in other cultures this is seen as an imposition. Child protection is paramount when working with children and their families. However, balancing protecting children from what individuals see as harmful and respecting the family's values can be very difficult when individual views on what is acceptable vary. Whether a child is suffering significant harm, or is at risk of suffering significant harm, is the key consideration. However, given the differences in what individuals may see as harmful, determining this can be problematic. This is one reason why those who work with children and young people should be aware of the processes, procedures and resources available to them related to child protection, and channels for discussing concerns and seeking advice on the best course of action.

As well as the principles of child protection that apply in all situations where staff work with children and their families, there are some specific issues to consider in safeguarding children who have complex and continuing health needs. Disabled children are more likely to experience abuse than children who are not disabled and may be less able to report this (Department of Health 2004a). Assumptions are sometimes made about the effects which a child's impairments have, which can mean that indicators of abuse are mistakenly attributed to these. Children who have complex health needs may have problems in reporting abuse. They are likely to have fewer outside contacts than their nondisabled peers and may have communication difficulties that make it hard for them to tell others what is happening to them. Receiving intimate personal care, often from a number of carers, may increase their risk of exposure to abusive behaviour, and make it more difficult for children to set and maintain boundaries with care staff. Dependence on an abusing carer can make it almost impossible for a child or young person to avoid abusive situations, or to tell anyone about the abuse. This is especially so if the abuser is a key person through whom they communicate or by whom they are usually accompanied when they are with other people. Society's negative attitudes to disabled children may also make it more difficult for them to find someone who will listen to them or believe them or believe them. Organisationally, a lack of appropriate services can leave disabled children and their families unsupported and physically and socially isolated which are risk factors for abuse and may mean that a child who has complex health needs is more at risk of abuse than another child would be (Department for Education and Skills 2006b).

Safeguards, which should be in place to prevent the abuse of children who have complex health needs or enable this to be identified at an early stage and acted on, are essentially the same as for nondisabled children and should include:

- Making it common practice for staff to aim to help children to make their wishes and feelings known.
- Ensuring that children receive appropriate personal, health and social education (including sex education).
- Making sure that all children know how to raise concerns, and giving them access to a range of adults with whom they can communicate.
- Children with communication impairments should have a means of being heard available to them at all times.
- Ensuring that guidelines exist and are adhered to, and that training exists and is accessed on: good practice in intimate care; working with children of the opposite sex; handling difficult behaviour; consent to treatment; anti-bullying strategies; sexuality and sexual behaviour amongst young people.

There should be close contact between families and staff, and a culture of openness on the part of service providers. There also needs to be an explicit commitment to, and understanding of, disabled children's safety and welfare among providers of services which are used by disabled children and amongst individuals who provide their day-to-day support.

The Children Act (Department of Health 2004b) establishes a duty on Local Authorities to make arrangements to promote co-operation between agencies in order to improve children's well-being, and a duty on key partners to take part in these arrangements. It also provides for pooling of resources in support of these arrangements. It requires that Local Authorities set up statutory Local Safeguarding Children Boards and that the key partners take part in these (Department of Health 2004b). These boards must also ensure that the specific needs of disabled children are addressed in safeguarding children protocols, including arranging advocacy services on their behalf where this may be beneficial.

Children and young people who have complex health needs have the same rights as other children and young people to be protected from harm. Protecting their rights in this respect may be more difficult, but is no less important, than it is for other children.

EQUALITY AND DISABILITY RIGHTS

Children and young people who have complex and continuing health needs have all the rights identified in The Disability Discrimination Act (HMSO 2005) and its predecessor the Disability Discrimination Act (HMSO 1995). This Act gives disabled people rights in the areas of: employment, education, access to goods, facilities, services, and buying or renting land or property. The Act has enabled minimum standards to be set so that disabled people have the right to expect to be able to use public transport easily, have access to everyday services, including shops, cafes, banks, cinemas and places of worship, health services and social services. It also means that they have the right to information about health and social services in a format that is accessible to them where it is reasonable for the service provider to provide it in that format. The Special Educational Needs and Disability Act 2001 (HMSO 2001) amended the Disability Discrimination Act 1995 to make it unlawful for education providers to discriminate against disabled pupils, students and adult learners, and to make sure disabled people are not disadvantaged in comparison to other people in relation to education.

The White Paper *Valuing People* (Department of Health 2001a) sets out a major programme to improve the life chances of all people with learning disabilities. Whilst not all children and young people who have complex and continuing health needs have learning disabilities, some may do, and their complex health needs do not detract from them having the same rights as other people with learning disabilities. *Valuing People* views independence as the expectation and states that services should, routinely, provide the support needed to enable people to make choices and express preferences about their day-to-day lives and to have these acted on. It identifies that enabling people with learning disabilities to be part of the mainstream is crucial if they are to be fully included in the life of the local community.

Children and young people who have complex and continuing health needs and their families have the rights identified in the Disability Discrimination Act (2005), and the Special Educational Needs and Disability Act (HMSO 2001) and the White Paper *Valuing People* (Department of Health 2001a). However, this does not always translate into them enjoying the same opportunities as other children, young people, and their families. What it does mean is that in some circumstances they can have legal recourse to seek improvement in the services which they receive and the facilities that are available to them, and can cite these documents in their arguments. Those who work with children and their families may be well placed to provide them with information on, or direct them to information on, their rights in this respect.

SUMMARY

Children and young people who have complex and continuing health needs have rights, as people, as children and as people who have disabilities. These rights are variously enshrined in policy, law and recommendations. The rights of the child and their well-being are paramount in all decisions that affect them.

Children and young people's rights include their right to be involved in decision making about them, and in decisions that affect them. The degree to which a child or young person is involved in decision making and the weight that is given to their views is affected by their age and level of understanding. Determining this, and the relative rights of parents and children or young people in decision making where their views are in conflict is not easy. However, the child or young person's ability to engage in decision making should not be confused with their physical abilities or their ability to communicate verbally.

Enabling children and young people to be involved in decision making is a responsibility of healthcare staff, but it is also their responsibility to provide them with support during this process. In addition, where children or young people are unused to being involved in decision making, they may be well placed to direct families to advocacy services and other relevant support mechanisms.

Protecting children, and in particular vulnerable children, is the responsibility of all healthcare staff. Those who work with children who have complex and continuing health needs should be aware of the mechanisms by which they can discuss concerns regarding child protection and the procedures that they should follow if abuse is suspected.

Children and young people who have complex health needs have certain rights as a result of the Disability Discrimination Act (HMSO 2005) and the Special Educational Needs and Disability Act (HMSO 2001). Staff may have useful role in supporting them in pursuing these rights.

Chapter 9
Ethical Issues Involved in Supporting Children, Young People and their Families

Working with children and young people who have complex and continuing health needs and their families can raise a number of debates or concerns for staff related to what is the ethically right course of action to follow. These can include what is considered to be beneficial or harmful for the individual or individuals with whom they work, how a person's best interests are determined, and how finite resources can be used for the good of all.

Such debates are not unique to working with children and young people who have complex and continuing health needs. However, there are some specific aspects of them that merit consideration when working with this group of people. This includes: debates over benefit and harm being complicated by the need to decide not only what is beneficial to the child or young person but the effect the decisions made in relation to them may have on their family; how decisions made in relation to one family impact on other service users; and how to make decisions on benefit and harm given the uncertainties that exist in many situations which involve people who have complex health needs. Working closely with the child, young person, and their family may also mean that it can be harder for staff to see situations completely objectively, or to see how what appears to one person or group of people to be beneficial could be viewed otherwise.

The staff who support children and young people who have complex health needs on a day-to-day basis may be involved in discussing their views on the available options for treatment, care and support with the child or young person, their family and other professionals. Understanding the different ways in which the main ethical principles underpinning healthcare provision may be interpreted and how they may be related to the decisions which have been made may therefore be useful.

MORALS AND ETHICS

Morals have been described as 'concerned with the principles of right and wrong behaviour' (Soanes et al. 2001). Ethics and morals are intrinsically linked, an ethic being defined as: 'a set of moral principles' (Soanes et al. 2001). Ethics might therefore be defined as the rules that distinguish what is deemed to be right conduct from that which is deemed to be wrong conduct.

A code of ethics makes explicit the stance on moral values and obligations of the profession to which they pertain (Nursing and Midwifery Council 2004). This essentially means that a code of ethics describes what the profession in question has deemed to be right or wrong conduct. Although the ethical principles to which nursing and other healthcare professions subscribe are ostensibly the same, each profession's interpretation of these and each individual professional's interpretation of these may differ. Thus, whilst healthcare professions and professionals all theoretically subscribe to the same moral and ethical principles, how these are viewed and enacted by professional groups and individuals may differ, despite the people concerned all believing that they are acting ethically.

Ethical and legal aspects of practice are often discussed together, but these are two different types of obligation. The moral or ethical stance that an individual or profession adopts may be different from the legal standards of a particular jurisdiction or laws of a country (McLelland 2006). Whilst healthcare professionals have an obligation, as citizens, to obey the law of the country they are in, doing so does not guarantee that they have behaved in accordance with their profession's code of ethics. Neither does following what an individual believes to be an ethically sound pathway personally or professionally guarantee that they do not break the law. Individual healthcare professionals are responsible for deciding whether or not to act lawfully and for justifying how their conduct meets the ethical requirements of their profession. Where such requirements are in conflict, the individual practitioner is required to weigh up and be able to justify the decisions that they make.

PROMOTING HEALTH

The promotion of health is seen as a moral imperative in healthcare, with actions which promote health considered moral and those which produce the opposite effect viewed as immoral (Wilmot 2003). This means that there is an ethical requirement for healthcare practitioners to promote health and to prevent ill health. However, determining whether or not this has been achieved requires health to be defined. There is no absolute consensus within healthcare professions on what constitutes health, or what the most important facet of health is. Thus, there are likley to be situations where there is a lack of complete agreement between professionals on what consititutes the ethically sound course of action in relation to promoting health.

Sullivan (2003) argues that in recent history the biomedical model of health has dominated healthcare in western society and led to health being seen as an objective biological fact, with cure of measurable physiological disease viewed as the optimum outcome. This has meant that interventions focused on the cure or reduction of physical ill health have been seen as the ethically or morally right aim of healthcare. However, a broader view of health, which includes the contributions of social, psychological, spiritual, cultural and emotional factors, is now acknowledged in healthcare (Royal College of Nursing 2003). This is a positive change, in regarding people as individuals, and seeing health and well-being holistically, but nevertheless means that debates related to the definition of health have to take into account a great deal more than the imperative to promote physical health.

What health means to individuals and what each individual sees as important in their health varies greatly. What one healthcare professional sees as good health, or the most important aspect of health, may be different from how another professional views this. What a healthcare professional sees as good health may not be the same as what a child, young person, or their parents perceive to be good health. A child who requires assisted ventilation is likely to see good health very differently from how a child who does not require assisted ventilation describes this. How a child defines health may be different from how their family describe health and from how healthcare providers view health. What individuals see as a priority within their health may also differ from how others would see their priorities. The moral or ethical imperative to promote health therefore requires more to be taken into account than simply taking measures to prevent or cure physiological disease processes or to minimise the physical effects of any disease or physical impairment. Health is a very complex and individual concept and as such no hard and fast rules over what consititues health, or the promotion thereof, can exist.

A further issue in working with children and young people who have complex health needs is that the imperative to promote health also requires consideration of how one person's state of health impacts on the state of health of others. For example, as Chapter 3 identifies, a child's state of health often has an effect on their parents' well-being, and the well-being of their siblings. Although, as identified in Chapter 8, the welfare of the child is paramount (Department of Health 2004b), the well-being of all children is paramount, and thus the well-being of the siblings of a child who has complex health needs, as well the well-being of the affected child, must be considered paramount. In addition, parent's state of health and well-being has the potential to impact on their children, and thus consideration of the well-being of parents is an important part of promoting the child's health and well-being.

Case study

Dione is 11. She requires CPAP at night and supplemental oxygen during the day. She is fed via a gastrostomy and is immobile. She has frequent seizures. Dione lives with her mother Grace, her father Josh, her sister Danielle and her brother Samuel. She has carers to support her at night, whilst she is at school, and on the way to and from school. However, the rest of the time her family manage her care.

Dione often becomes very irritable during the day, and her care needs are becoming harder to manage because of this. She says she feels very tired and gets more headaches than she previously did. It is thought that she might benefit from some respiratory support during the day. However, whether this should be commenced is under debate related to whether it will improve her quality of life, whether it is right to engage in this level of intervention given her underlying lung damage and level of disability, and whether this is an appropriate use of resources.

Grace feels that it would be best for Dione to try using CPAP during the day. She believes that it would make her feel better, and make her more positive about life and more co-operative over things like getting dressed, and being changed. She also believes that Dione's quality of life would be improved and she would once again enjoy things she used to. However, she is concerned that Dione will need closer observation and more care than she does now, and wonders how this will be achieved without impacting on her brother and sister. She is aware that they might need 24-hour assistance, which, whilst it might be helpful, might also be very intrusive for the family as a whole. Equally, she worries that since Dione has become less well her siblings have suffered, because she is not the sister they knew, and because she has to spend more time with Dione because of her disinclination for the care activities which she needs. If Dione was better, even if it meant more intervention, and less privacy for the family as a whole, it might make life easier for her siblings.

Grace thinsk that providing CPAP during the day may increase Dione's life expectancy and reduce the number of chest infections which she gets. However, her main concern is her quality of life, and the quality of life of the whole family.

The requirement to promote health, whilst undeniably an ethical requirement in healthcare, is therefore not a simple task and not one that will always be clear-cut in terms of the best course of action. Whilst there are few easy answers in ethical decision making in healthcare, there are ethical principles that can be used to guide and inform practitioners.

ETHICAL PRINCIPLES

Beauchamp and Childress (2001) describe four principles of medical ethics that form one of the most widely used frameworks for debating healthcare ethics. These four principles are beneficence, nonmaleficence, autonomy and justice.

Beneficence

Beneficence is concerned with the provision of benefit and is linked with non-maleficence, which is concerned with preventing harm (Wilmot 2003). In order to act ethically, healthcare staff should always act in a way which is beneficial for service users. However, as described previously, individual views on what is beneficial or harmful varies. What one person considers beneficial another may consider harmful. What is physically beneficially may be detrimental to an individual's social or psychological well-being. Where a child or young person has complex health needs, it may be that an intervention which has some benefits also has some negative outcomes or risks. Thus, an intervention or action by a member of healthcare staff or a decision regarding healthcare may not be wholly beneficial or harmful, but rather the balance of benefit and harm must be sought in which the likely outcome is weighed in favour of benefit rather than harm.

Where children, young people, and their families are concerned, who will benefit and at what cost to others may also need to be considered. For example, parents may have to make decisions in which the benefit to the child who has complex health needs, their siblings and the parents themselves have to be included and the relative weight that will be afforded to the cost versus benefit analysis of each situation (Menahem and Grimwade 2003; Hewitt-Taylor 2007).

For many families, this type of decision making has to happen almost every day, as a part of their life, in small everyday events as well as in major life decisions. The impact that previous decisions have on current decisions, the history of decision making in the family, and how inevitable differences of opinion have been negotiated will contribute to ongoing decision making. These are not necessarily decisions to which healthcare staff will have been privy, but are considerations of which they should be aware because they may influence what families see as beneficial or harmful, the pre-existing assumptions and agreed value systems which they bring to any discussion and the position from which family members who may have differences of opinion are negotiating.

Case study

Julia is six years old. She was born at 24 weeks gestation and has residual lung damage, which means that she needs CPAP at night. She also has cerebral palsy, hearing problems, and epilepsy.

Julia lives at home with her mother, Rosie. Rosie's partner left soon after Julia was born. His opinion was that treatment should have been withdrawn during the neonatal period. He could see no benefit to his daughter, his partner or himself in continued intervention.

Rosie always felt that Julia should have the chance to be treated. The outcome of their difference of opinion was that Rosie's partner declined any further input into Rosie or Julia's lives, as it was not what he had chosen.

Julia recently developed a chest infection, and Rosie was very prompt and concerned in her choices of treatment. She explained: 'I do get things started very quickly. I am that pushy parent. But my whole life, since Julia was born, has been fighting for her rights. Her right for a chance to live. So, yes, I do start from the position that I am defending her, because I have always had to. I have always had people wanting me to give up on her. I have always had to fight her corner.'

Nonmaleficence

Nonmaleficence concerns avoiding the causation of harm, and is therefore closely linked to the requirement to do good: the ethical stance being that healthcare staff should act in a way which is beneficial to service users and does them no harm. Like the requirement to do good, this nonetheless leaves open to debate what constitutes harm, to whom, and the balance of benefit and harm for all people concerned in decision making.

Case study

Belinda is 11. She has difficulty swallowing, is fed via a gastrostomy, and is meant to only take sips of fluids. However, one of her pleasures in life has been eating, joining in family meals, having lunch with her friends at school, and the social interactions around food. She still chooses to eat, small amounts, but enough to taste and join in events. She and her family are aware that this poses a risk to her, but have decided that this is important to her overall quality of life.

Belinda relies on someone being prepared to assist her: to get her food, cut it up, and place it in front of her. Her parents do this for her when they are present, but some staff refuse to do so because it is physically harmful to her.

Respect for Autonomy

As discussed in Chapter 8, respect for autonomy is currently high on healthcare agendas (Joffe et al. 2003; Sullivan 2003). However, this has not always been the case. Kennedy (2003) identifies that, in healthcare, patients' best interests were traditionally unquestioningly judged by medical staff and that it would have been considered unreasonable, and even harmful, to impose the burden of decision making on them. As discussed in Chapter 8, this view is now generally seen as unhelpful and it has been suggested that reducing a person's autonomy reduces their well-being. A failure to respect autonomy is now therefore generally considered to also mean that the moral requirement to promote health is not met. Failure to fulfil the obligation to promote autonomy may therefore be linked to failing to comply with the principles of beneficence and nonmalificence as this is not beneficial, and may be harmful (Kennedy 2003; Wilmot 2003).

The moral value of autonomy is also linked to the moral imperative to promote health insofar as ill health tends to decrease an individual's autonomy (Wilmot 2003). The concepts of health and autonomy are thus intertwined: assisting an individual to achieve health may improve their autonomy, and enabling a person to become autonomous may assist them to achieve good health. However, if returning health and therefore autonomy is a moral imperative, there could be an argument that a temporary infringement of an individual's autonomy is morally permissible if this has the aim of improving their health and therefore by implication ultimately their autonomy. This argument has been used as a part of the justification for healthcare professionals engaging in decision making on behalf of service users (Wilmot 2003). However, Wilmot (2003) suggests that this is not generally a justifiable approach and that other issues are usually involved when healthcare staff choose to make decisions on behalf of people who have not been deemed incapable of exercising their autonomy. In addition, the assumption that decision making by another person is acceptable relies on the person making such decisions knowing what the individual in question considers to constitute health, their priorities and values. As previous chapters have described, this is unlikely to be the case in the vast majority of healthcare encounters. As discussed in

Chapter 8, where a child has complex health needs, the requirement to promote autonomy may be complicated, but the complexity of achieving this does not negate the ethical requirement to do so.

Case study

Georgia is 14. She has difficulty speaking, and uses signing and picture cards to communicate. She was recently advised that it would be beneficial for her to have a new medication to treat her seizures. She was not given any information about this except that it is a new drug which will help her.

Georgia tried to ask, via her carers and mother, what the drug is, how it will improve her seizures, and what the common side effects are. However, although her mother is very good at communicating with Georgia, she does not like to question medical staff.

Georgia has now started to receive the medication, which is administered via her gastrostomy. She thinks her seizures may have improved slightly but also thinks that the drug makes her feel sleepy all day. However, what she feels very unhappy about is that she realises that she has very little say in her treatment, or her life.

Justice

Justice is concerned with distributing benefits, risks and costs fairly. The aim of justice in healthcare should be to provide all individuals with equal access to what might be considered a basic need, such as health (Wilmot 2003). Grace (2001) identifies that actions taken in relation to one person necessarily have implications beyond the person to whom they are directed and thus the ethical principles of preventing harm, doing good and promoting autonomy have to be seen alongside the requirement for justice. However, this is not easy to achieve as it includes consideration of local and national resource allocation for a range of health related conditions and interventions (Fletcher and Buka 1999; Bridges et al. 2001).

A further difficulty is that because what health means for individuals varies greatly, what a basic level of good health will mean also varies. The complexity of achieving justice in healthcare provision includes providing equal access to all, but also acknowledging that for each individual what needs they would want to have met, and how they would want these needs to be met varies. Provision which would be of equal value to all or of equal benefit to all is therefore extremely difficult to determine. A wider view of health than the biomedical model creates the need to include all aspects of health in decision making, and to consider the range of options which individuals might find beneficial to their health. Whilst this more holistic view of health represents a more person-centered approach to healthcare than the biomedical model, it also makes debating and achieving justice in healthcare resource allocation more complex.

As well as the complexity of deciding on how healthcare needs can be equally met, the ever developing capacity to manage complex health problems has increased dilemmas over resource allocation and rationing of services (Boosfeld and O'Toole 2000; Poses 2003). The resources for a health service which is free at the point of delivery, such as the National Health Service, cannot meet all the needs which everyone has as soon as would be ideal. In order to determine how resources should be used, utilitarian principles are often used or described as being used. In this approach, the outcome of an action justifies it's means and the principle of the most productive use of resources and the greatest good for the greatest number is often cited (Draper and Sorell 2002). Using this approach, justice would require that healthcare resources be used in a way which creates the greatest good for the greatest number of people or uses resources the most productively overall. However, this does not simplify the debate on resource allocation, as it still requires what is good and what is productive to be determined. Given the range of views on what is good or beneficial, this is difficult, if not impossible, to achieve across populations.

Attempts to achieve justice in decision making about national resources can be approached by central decision making regarding the value of various uses of healthcare funding. For example, one of the remits of the National Institute for Health and Clinical Excellence (NICE) is for experts employed by NICE to consider whether various treatments, interventions or technologies are a valid use of resources based on the best overall use of the available funds (NICE 2005). However, one of the problems with this approach is that such a body cannot take into account individual preferences or perceptions of benefit and priorities. Whilst NICE consult widely, and include organisations which represent service users as well as professionals in their decision-making processes, decisions still have to be made on the basis the current best evidence of clinical and cost effectiveness, and as perceived by the team of reviewers. This often means that the evidence related to cure of disease or relief of physical symptoms is the focus (Hewitt-Taylor 2006).

In contrast with the principles of utilitarianism, deontological principles judge an action solely on the benefit of its own outcome, isolated from broader consequences. Whilst this places the individual, and their well-being, centrally, it may be considered incompatible with the complexities of modern healthcare provision in which decisions made in relation to one person will inevitably impact on the resources available for others. This view may therefore be seen as unjust, because it will inevitably lead to inequality in provision. However, for practitioners faced with individual need, this may be a difficult stance to avoid. It may also be difficult not to adopt this approach when seeking to provide support that acknowledges the importance of respecting individual priorities, values and choices.

The four ethical principles do not, therefore, provide an easy answer to debates related to the ethical issues associated with the support that is provided for children and young people who have complex health needs and their families. In addition, the principles are not stand alone features, but need to be considered together. Lenton (2006) suggests that all of the principles are equally important and that the assessment of best interests involves a complex examination of all the potentially conflicting influences of these four principles. When working with children and their families, how the implications of one principle being enacted for one person impacts on the fulfillment of that or another principle for another member of the family, and other members of society has to be taken into account. This means that very few, if any, easy answers exist and staff who work with children, young people, and their families are well advised to be aware of the complexity that decision making can involve.

Case study

James manages a team of nurses employed to support children who have complex and continuing health needs and their families. The budget and staffing establishment for the team is set, and as more children and young people are being referred to them it is becoming increasingly difficult to cover the support required. When the team was set up, three years ago, they provided 24-hour support for two children who required assisted ventilation, and short-break care once a month for three other children. They now have a caseload of three children who require 24-hour assisted ventilation, three who require CPAP at night, and four who require short-break care. They also have occasional input into the support of three children who have gastrostomies and require oxygen during the day. James explains how:

'When the team was set up, we could be very flexible, we could juggle things to meet the families' needs, and we could try to match staff really closely with the family's needs, see who got on best with whom, what hours suited everyone. We still try to do that, but we are now stretched across more than double our original workload. It means we have had to cut down on the extras, the occasional extra twilight shift so that someone's Mum can get a break, or a child could go to a special event, or stay after school to do something. The short breaks are much stricter now too, we have to book them well in advance and we have very little flexibility, because the resources are so stretched. It is hard on families, because you want to give them the best, but you have to give them all the best, and the pot of money is having to be stretched across more families. You can't give it all to one and then say to the next "Sorry, nothing left for you!"

DUTIES OF HEALTHCARE PROFESSIONALS

The four ethical principles discussed above are often accompanied or appended by discussion of four additional rules of healthcare, or duties which healthcare professionals have. These are: veracity, privacy, confidentiality and fidelity (Beauchamp and Childress 2001).

Veracity

Veracity, or truth telling, is based on the principle that respect is owed to others (Beauchamp and Childress 2001). Respect, as Chapters 2–5 identify, should be a mainstay of the relationship between healthcare staff, children, young people and their families. Telling the truth is a part of respecting a person and therefore a part of the respect owed to children, young people and their families. Veracity also influences the achievement of autonomy, because unless a person is told the truth they cannot make a truly informed choice, as they will not have received accurate information on which to base this. If a person cannot rely on being told the truth by another person, they cannot trust them and thus the requirement for fidelity, or trust, is also affected by the fulfilment of the obligation to be truthful.

There have nonetheless been suggestions that there are times when the requirement for truth telling can be overridden by other concerns in healthcare, for example, when healthcare staff believe that the truth could be iatrogenic. However, if individuals are seen as autonomous, it is not the right of another person to decide that to tell them the truth would be harmful to justify giving them inaccurate or deceptive information, or withholding information from them (Da Silva et al. 2003). It has nonetheless been identified that whilst healthcare staff generally oppose lying, there are many ways in which staff have been found to avoid telling the truth (Tuckett 1998; Kirklin 2007). This includes using metaphors that obscure the truth or failing to give sufficiently powerful or revealing information in their discussions with service users (Kirklin 2007). Although such tactics may enable staff to avoid overtly lying, they do not constitute truth telling as the intention is to deliberately conceal the truth, or the full truth, from another person. The requirement to tell the truth means that staff have a responsibility to ensure that messages are conveyed in a way that enables the recipient to understand the information and which does not have the intention of misrepresenting the facts or another person's interpretation of these.

Case study

Hannah is four. She was born prematurely, has very limited mobility, is fed via a gastrostomy, and has CPAP at night. Her mother, Olivia, recalls:

'They said I would have support all night, to manage her CPAP, so that I could get some sleep. I do, but what they didn't explain was that for them 'night' is 10 pm til 6 am. It is good to have that help, but I agreed to take her home thinking I could get some sleep. By the time they arrive, and you tell them any changes, it's half ten at the earliest, then by the time I get to bed, the earliset I can ever go to sleep is 11. I have to be up at 5 to get ready to take over again, because they leave at 6. So it isn't really "night care" like I was promised. I was told that they had employed staff to provide that night care, and it turned out they hadn't got enough staff, it was about 50% agency staff, who were fine, but it meant that I had different people every night for a while. I also didn't realise that if someone went off sick they couldn't replace them, so it was down to me.

'I was told I would have support from the nurse specialist for gastrostomies, and I have seen her once, when I asked to. So, I suppose you could say she is there if I need her, but I was given the impression that she would routinely be involved, not that she would only be available if I made a specific request. I was also told that I would get some short-break care, and that hasn't really happened, because although Hannah is eligible, there isn't any available. So, although nothing I was told was actually untrue, it just isn't quite as I was led to believe. I would still have taken her home, because she is my daughter and I want her home, but I didn't really know the facts when I said yes. On bad days, I think "They lied to me, to get us out of hospital!"'

Privacy

All people have a right to privacy, both in their individual life and in healthcare settings. This right exists by means of the European Convention on Human Rights (1948, article 12) (Council of Europe 1950) and the Universal Declaration on Bioethics and Human Rights (McLelland 2006). Privacy and the challenges which can be encountered in achieving this when supporting children and young people who have complex health needs have been alluded to in other chapters. However, it is an obligation, legally, and professionally, for health-care staff to protect the privacy of those with whom they work. Where staff work with families in their homes, they are likely to have access to a greater amount of private information than in other settings, and the privacy of this information as well as the child, young person and family's personal privacy and privacy of healthcare information should be respected.

Confidentiality

Confidentiality in a professional relationship (such as that between a health-care professional and service user) is part of privacy, and as such is protected by the right to privacy. However, the right which service users have to confi-dentiality related to healthcare information imposes an obligation on persons who obtain such information in healthcare relationships not to disclose this information (McLelland 2006).

The prime reason for not disclosing personal information without consent is that the person concerned may not want it to be disclosed. Just as individuals have a right to self-determination in every other area of their lives, who should have access to their personal information and how it should be used should be their decision (McLelland 2006). The person who owns the information (ie the person to whom it pertains) is in the best position to understand the impli-cations of information being disclosed and therefore protect their interests by deciding with whom the information should be shared. Individuals deciding who will have information about them, and for what purpose, is an intrinsic part of them deciding about and taking responsibility for their own lives, and others respecting this is a part of respecting their right to autonomy (McLelland 2006). Respect for confidentiality is a fundamental part of respect for individ-uals and a part of the ethical requirement to respect individual's autonomy.

There may nonetheless, exceptionally, be circumstances where the require-ment to respect confidentiality can be overridden. This includes situations where the person who owns the information requests or consents to this, statutory exceptions (such as the notification of certain infectious diseases), where child protection is an issue, and in the public interest (Dimond 2005). Any disclosure of confidential information requires healthcare professionals to have regard for its necessity, proportionality and any attendant risks (McLel-land 2006). Where information is given to a healthcare professional with the expectation that it will be confidential, the person must be warned if this is not likely to be the case. This includes disclosure of information which children share with their parents (Dimond 2005).

> ## Case study
>
> Jocelyn is eight years old. She goes to mainstream school, and has previously been happy and achieved well there. However, last week her carer, Adah, who escorts her to and from school, noticed that she is very quiet after school, and unwilling to discuss her day in the way she was previously. She asked Jocelyn whether there was a problem at school, and eventually Jocelyn said that some of the other girls were being 'mean' to her. Adah talked to her about this and asked if she would like to talk to her mother or teachers. Jocelyn said she did not want to, because her mother would only worry, and if the teachers became involved the other children might 'get worse'. Adah felt that it would be better if Joceyln's mother or school were informed, and said that she would be prepared to be with her during discussions if she wanted this. However, she promised that she would not speak to anyone without Jocelyn's permission. She also told Jocelyn that other people might ask her if she was OK, and that, in this case, she would not lie, but would ask them to ask Jocelyn.
>
> The next day, Jocelyn's teacher asked Adah if there was anything wrong with Jocelyn, as she seemed very withdrawn. Adah suggested that the teacher ask Jocelyn because only she would know how she was feeling, and what she wanted to tell other people about.

FIDELITY

A tacit understanding exists within the relationship between healthcare professionals and service users that healthcare professionals will be trustworthy. The European Standards on Confidentiality and Privacy in Healthcare identify that the relationship between the healthcare professional and the patient is, or should be, one of 'fidelity' or 'trust' (McLelland 2006). This includes healthcare staff demonstrating trustworthiness in information giving and fulfilling the trust that their privacy and right to confidentiality will be maintained.

Fidelity is concerned with faithfully maintaining the duty to care, even in difficult circumstances, and fulfilling the trust which people place in healthcare staff. Thus, breach of any part of the duty of care or of any ethical requirement can be seen as a breach of fidelity.

RESPONSIBILITY

Debates over medical ethics often emphasise the need to safeguard the autonomy of service users, but fail to acknowledge that autonomy goes hand in hand with responsibility (Draper and Sorell 2002). Promoting and respecting individual's autonomy does not mean that support or caring should be withdrawn from the decision-making process. However, a person who makes decisions for themsleves must also take responsiblity for these. After a focus on medical professionals' obligations to service users for most of the twentieth century, there is now a growing interest in the responsibility which service users have. Appropriately informed autonomous individuals are responsible for the outcomes of their decisions in relation to their health as much as in any other area of life.

Children, young people and their parents should take responsibility for their decisions, and healthcare staff should provide accurate and full information to enable them to make such decisions. However, the speed with which medicine and technology advance, and the complexity and rarity of the medical problems which some children and young people have means that certainty over the outcomes of treatment or interventions is very difficult to achieve. The options that will be available to them in years to come are also often largely unknown. In addition, the nature of some children and young people's needs means that options for treatment or care for them are not well established or tested. The likely outcomes of interventions, treatment or care are therefore often uncertain. However, experts and lay people alike tend to desire certainty rather than acknowledgement of ambiguity or the relative but uncertain nature of risks in all areas of life, including healthcare (English 2005).

Whilst certainty is attractive, and consistency of information giving by professionals important for staff, where it does not exist, truthful and clear discussion of the knowns, unknowns and relative risks of any treatment or intervention being considered is necessary. Where decision making must be based on the balance of benefit versus harm, rather than absolute or definite benefit, professionals should be aware that this is difficult for many children, young people and their families. Autonomy in decision making should not be equated with abdication of the duty of care by healthcare staff. Rather, it makes supportive and nonjudgemental facilitation of decision making imperative, with support available after the event as children, young people and their families live with and review their decision making, often in the light of new evidence.

SUMMARY

One of the difficulties in ethical decision making is weighing up the many facets of the ethical principles that should underpin healthcare provision, and applying these to children, young people and their families in circumstances where certainty is elusive. However, an individual should never be knowingly engaged in a course of action that causes harm unless the benefit outweighs the harm. Those supporting children and their families should be aware that what is harmful and beneficial in individual cases is usually best determined by the individuals themselves, but also the complexity of balancing what will be beneficial for one individual with what will be beneficial for another.

It may not always be possible to provide everything an individual or family wants, or needs, and the reality of finite resources will always be an issue in publicly-funded healthcare which is free at the point of delivery. Truthful dialogue between healthcare providers and service users about the realities of resource availability should occur, so that families know the choices which they have, and limits of these, and can make autonomous decisions within what is available. Although autonomy brings with it responsibility, a supportive and compassionate environment should be created for children, young people and their families during and after decision making processes.

Chapter 10
Organisational Issues

When children and young people who have complex and continuing health-care needs live at home, they and their families often require support which involves a range of organisations and professional groups (Noyes 2006b). This chapter explores some of the elements of support that children, young people and their families may require, and how this support should be managed in order to provide a high quality of service.

SUPPORT

There are a range of activities that are considered to contribute to providing support for children, young people and their families. One aspect of this is information being made available to them. Parents have described how important it for them to have easy access to a full range of accurate, consistent and timely information (Redmond and Richardson 2003). This includes information about: the child or young person's condition and prognosis, treatment and care options that exist, services which are available for them, how to obtain referrals to services, the state benefits and allowances which they may be able to claim, and support groups which may be useful for them. Healthcare professionals may not be able to give families information regarding all these issues, but should be able to refer or direct families to other individuals, agencies or organisations where necessary.

Whilst healthcare staff are not expected to have answers to all the questions that children, young people and their families have, or information about every aspect of their care and support, even in their area of expertise, providing as full information as is available, and being honest over unknowns, is important (Hewitt-Taylor 2007). Whilst information should be truthful, full and accurate, it also needs to be delivered sensitively and in a way that does not overload the recipient at any one time. It should be delivered in a manner that takes into account the amount and enormity of some of the information which is provided, but which is not misleading or reductionist of what are complex issues. Children, young people and their families should have opportunities to revisit and develop information, and to ask questions and discuss individual concerns over time, not only when the information is given to them. The way in which information is delivered, like all aspects of support should indicate caring concern but also respect for children, young people and their families, and their right to make their own decisions (Hewitt-Taylor 2007).

Case study

Karen is 13. She was diagnosed as having Rett Syndrome when she was five years old. Her parents, Alan and Wendy, describe how 'A lot of things we have just found out as we went along. At first, we were told: "She has Rett Syndrome. That's why she has developmental delay." That was about it. We were told she would get worse, not better, but no one explained what worse meant, that she would start having seizures, that she would stop being able to eat. We moved house when she was six. If we had known how she would be, we might have thought ahead a bit more, and had the ceiling hoist and everything put in then. Instead, we moved, and then had to have the house ripped out around us. Some people seem to think we should have known. We did know . . . we did know she couldn't walk, but we had never seen a 13 year old who was disabled before. Or not lived with them, not seen how you have to lift them, how many things you have to think about, so we didn't think: "Oh, we'll need a ceiling track hoist, let's get that put in." We just moved to a bungalow. So, we did have information, but not really enough about what we should think about. What it would mean.'

Emotional support is important for some children, young people and their families, but there is evidence that there is a relative lack of this type of support and that its availability depends a great deal on individual care staff's inclination and skills in providing this (Abbott et al. 2005). Parents whose children who have complex health needs often find peer support groups very valuable, because they enable them to discuss their experiences with other people who are in a similar situation. For some families, this is the most important and valid mechanism for personal or emotional support, because other families are able to understand their situation better than professionals, and to empathise with them (Kerr and McIntosh 2000; Hewitt-Taylor 2007).

Support groups may also be a good mechanism for children, young people and their families to access information that is not widely available. They also often produce information that is presented in a way which is meaningful to parents and addresses issues that are important for them to know about and consider in everyday life. Internet support groups may be very useful, especially given the difficulties which families whose children have complex needs can encounter in going out and meeting other people (Hewitt-Taylor 2007). Providing families with information about such groups may be a very important part of information giving, and may be a very valuable way of providing them with access to emotional support. Some examples of such groups can be seen in the Appendix.

Families may also need practical assistance, for example, help with obtaining supplies and equipment, and with the child or young person's care. This type of support can vary in duration from a few hours a week to the provision of 24-hour support. The amount and type of support which is provided needs to be tailored to the needs of the child and family, balancing intrusion into the family's life and home, as described in Chapter 5, with assistance. It is useful for service providers to discuss with families how they think this balance can best be managed at the planning stage of support, and for agreements to be made over the role of staff who are in the family home, and the responsibilities and expectations of both parties. There should also be a clear mechanism for how and when the level and type of support provided will be reviewed (Widdas et al. 2005).

Condliffe (2006) identifies that providing children and their families with support should have the aim of enabling them to achieve what they consider to be good quality of life. As Chapter 2 and 3 describe, what individuals consider to be good quality of life varies. In order for support to enable individual children, young people, and their families to achieve good quality of life, it must therefore be tailored to what this means to them, their preferences and lifestyle (as far as is possible within the constraints of resources). The level of satisfaction which service users have with healthcare provision includes more than whether services are medically or technically competent, and meet an individual's physical needs. It is affected by whether individuals feel that they and their personal identity are valued (Coyle 1999). A service that provides support in a way which meets a child or young person's physical needs, but does not take into account their preferences, priorities and identity or see them as people and as a part of their family is unlikely to enhance their life or make them feel valued and respected as people. In order to provide high-quality support, service providers therefore need to consider what the child or young person and their family as a whole need, and to tailor services to enable them to enjoy quality of life, as individuals and as a family, as far as is possible.

DETERMINING WHAT IS NEEDED

Need is defined as: 'To require because it is essential, or very important' (Soanes et al. 2001). However, because what individuals define as quality of life and their personal and family circumstances vary, what each child and family will need to assist them to achieve quality of life will be different. What professionals assess service users as requiring may not be what the person concerned wants, or sees as their need. The expectation is that children, young people, and their families should be included in decisions which are made about them (Department of Health 2004a). This should apply equally to decisions about the support that they receive as to other decisions, as only they can know what is important to them and what is likely to be helpful and supportive input.

Whilst the principle that the views of children, young people and their families should guide the way in which need is assessed and support organised is not disputed and is the ideal, this can be complicated. One difficulty in achieving this is defining what is absolute need, and what is something which families would like, but do not absolutely need, and how far finite budgets can meet all needs. Whilst individuals may perceive that they have a need, and professionals may agree with this, there is, as identified in Chapter 9, a finite amount of staffing and funding for what is rapidly becoming an infinite demand for healthcare provision. Thus, whilst families should be central to decision-making processes, some of their needs may not be able to be met. This may require very frank discussions regarding availability of resources and choices which have to be made, and the priorities that families have. Whilst the ultimate provision of support will always have to be within finite funding, children, young people and their families' priorities and needs should dictate how this funding is spent. If not, the risk is that money will be spent, but good quality support not achieved.

Not all family members may agree on what they need, or what they most need. Where there is discord between members of the family, healthcare staff have to be very clear about who has parental responsibility for the child or young person in question, the weight that should be given to the child or young person's views and their parents' views (as discussed in Chapter 8). They may also need to clarify to families that resolution of differences of opinion on their preferences are their responsibility. Whilst healthcare professionals may be able to facilitate family discussions, they may need to clarify the limits of their responsibility in this respect and be able to direct families to additional support services if appropriate.

Whilst all families will have different requirements for support, and levels at which the intrusion which having staff in their home creates will outweigh the assistance which they provide, they will also have different thresholds for seeking support or seeing this as their right or need. Although some families may perceive that they need more support than can realistically be offered, some expect very little and may need assistance to avail themselves of support which might be beneficial to them. One of the methods by which staff may be able to support families is by encouraging those who would like support to articulate this and to appreciate it as their right. Respectful direction in enabling families to gain support may be invaluable in some cases. If families do not, at any given time, want assistance, or a particular type of help, to which they are entitled, it is useful for them to have information on mechanisms by which this can be sought at a later stage if desired.

Case study

Rosemary, aged three, has very limited mobility, is fed via a gastrostomy, and requires CPAP 24 hours a day. Her mother, Pat, has always cared for her at home, except during brief periods of hospitalisation. Pat also has another daughter, Janine, who is five. Pat has always had night carers from 9 pm until 7 am to assist her with Rosemary's care. However, she has never had any day care or short-break care.

Recently, one of her carers asked Pat if she felt she needed more support. Pat admitted that she did find caring for both her daughters tiring and that she never had enough time to spend with Janine. However, she also felt that as she had assistance at night she was 'luckier than some' and did not like to ask for extra help. Her carer explained that she did have a right to ask for more help, for example, short-break care, and that whilst no guarantees could be made, this request would be reasonable. Pat said that she would think about it.

The next week, Pat asked the carer whom she should contact about being assessed for more support. A year later, Pat has four weekends a year short-break care, and Rosemary has five hours a week of support funded by social services to enable Pat to spend more time with Janine.

JOINED-UP ASSESSMENT

It is likely that families whose children have complex health needs will have input from Local Authorities, Local Education Authorities, Primary Care Trusts and NHS Trusts. They will often also be involved with a range of professionals within these services (Department of Health 2004a). For support to be effective, these agencies and the staff within them need to work effectively together.

The process of working together should ideally begin at or before the point of assessment so that the child or young person and their family's needs are comprehensively, holistically and consistently assessed. This should also reduce the need for repetitive information giving which can be intrusive for families and very time-consuming for them and service providers (Department of Health 2001a; Boddy et al. 2006). To assist professionals from a range of services to assess a child or young person and their family's needs, and to improve the consistency of assessment, frameworks have been devised which can be used across disciplines and services, such as the Common Assessment Framework (Department for Education and Skills 2006a).

As well as avoiding duplication of information, the Common Assessment Framework aims to help practitioners to develop a shared understanding of a child or young person's needs and to reduce delays in assessment and communication between services. This should mean that children, young people and their families can gain earlier access to the services that they need (Boddy et al. 2006; Condliffe 2006). Although the Common Assessment Framework does not specifically address the needs of children and young people who have complex and continuing health needs, it may be useful to incorporate this or a similar document within a joined-up assessment, as a tool for gathering baseline information about the child or young person and their family's needs in a format which all services can use.

Children and young people's needs and those of their families are likely to change over time. This may be because their health changes, because their needs change as they get older, because the family's circumstances change, or because their priorities alter. Mechanisms for assessment therefore need to be ongoing, not a one-off event (Elston 2003). Like initial assessment, ongoing assessment and evaluation of provision should be holistic, collaborative, and well-co-ordinated.

COLLABORATIVE WORKING

Once the child or young person's needs have been assessed, agencies need to work together to support them and their family. The Department of Health (2004a) suggest that disabled children have contact with an average of 10 different professionals and have in excess of 20 hospital visits per year. Within this, families are likely to have input from nurses who provide them with day-to-day support, specialist nurses, physiotherapists, occupational therapists, dieticians, medical staff, teachers, learning support assistants, portage workers, and social workers. This can mean that as well as having frequent professional visitors in their homes, families are overwhelmed by a range of appointments, plans and decisions.

Close liaison and co-ordination between all the services which are involved with the child and their family is essential if the amount of intrusion into their lives and unnecessary wasted time because of duplication of discussion and decision making is to be avoided (Craft 2004; Kirk and Glendinning 2004; Heaton et al. 2005; Hewitt-Taylor 2007). If there is no system which ensures that services are co-ordinated parents are often left with the role of co-ordinator of services, views and decisions, which can be very stressful, time consuming and can almost negate the benefit of the services provided (Hewitt-Taylor 2007).

Case study

Sally's son, Toby, is two. He is fed via a gastrostomy, has a tracheostomy and requires CPAP. He is seen by a paediatrician, a gastroenterologist, a dietician, a respiratory consultant, a respiratory nurse specialist, a cardiologist, a cardiac nurse specialist, a physiotherapist, an occupational therapist, a neurologist, a speech and language therapist, a portage worker, the health visitor and a specialist health visitor. Sally also occasionally needs to see her GP if Toby has any minor health problems. Sally has a carer to look after Toby at night. She also has one five-hour slot of daytime support each week.

Sally explains: 'I spend very little time actually with Toby. I spend all day with him, but I have that much to organise and do related to his medical needs that I don't get to do things with him. I have to get him to and from appointments, then wait to see people because they always run late. Going to appointments is a nightmare, because I have to take masses of stuff: the CPAP and suction machine and feeding tubes, feeds or water, syringes for that, any medication he needs, a spare trache tube, and nappies and wipes. Because they always run so late I have to take things to amuse him as well. I have to have a carer with me, or my Mum, because otherwise getting us and everything we need to appointments is impossible. All my carer time gets used up on appointments. Then there are the ones who come here, which is great because we don't have to get organised to go out, and we don't have to carry everything with us, but we have to be in and I have to make sure I have hoovered or tidied up and everything looks a bit respectable. They always say: "Oh, don't worry about us." But I don't want them going away saying "God, she lives in a tip." The other day, I had an appointment at the hospital at 10, then another one back here at 2, and we only got back just about by 1. That does annoy me about them being so late all the time, because it's not very respectful, to your life, is it? They do assume I have nothing else to do all day but wait around for them.

'Then the Health Visitor wanted to call round. I had to tell her no that day, because somewhere in all that Toby needs to have a sleep, and just some time to be with me. But cancelling her was another phone call. It may not seem a lot, but I have so many things to do. Calls about prescriptions, supplies, feeds, and then I have to be in when those all arrive. Phone calls to rearrange appointments that are at the same time but in different departments because they don't talk to each other, they just send me an appointment.

'When I see people, they all have a slightly different take on things, or different plans, so I have to chase that up and say: "Well, the respiratory consultant said . . ." so the neuro one says "Oh well, I don't think so." So I am pig in the middle trying to sort out their arguments and get them to talk to each other. They usually don't quite agree, or want to find out what the others think about their ideas, and then they say they'll write to each other or call each other, but they don't get back to me. So here I am not knowing what to do, because one says one thing and one says another. Then I am chasing results, or chasing letters I need, or forms I need signed. In between, I have the things Toby actually needs doing, his feeds, his suction, his CPAP, all his usual care … and I can't answer the phone when I'm doing suction, or setting up his feed, but they get really sniffy if I say: "Well when are you going to phone me, because I can't just be standing by waiting." I think because I don't work, I 'just' look after Toby they think I am sitting around all day waiting for a phone call.'

Where many disciplines work together, multi agency and multidisciplinary working is inevitable. What is required to enable children and their families to have effective support and achieve optimum quality of life is for all the disciplines and agencies involved to work effectively together, with a focus on the child or young person and their family's needs (Department of Health 2004a). There is considerable discussion over the terms 'multidisciplinary' 'inter professional' and 'interdisciplinary' (Atwal and Caldwell 2006). Regardless of nomenclature, what is essential for children and their families is that the variety of agencies, services and professionals involved in supporting them work in a cohesive and well-coordinated manner. This includes them having clarity over who is responsible for each aspect of support, whom they should communicate with regarding each aspect of provision, and assurance that there is an agreed goal and plan towards which all services are working.

Good communication within and between teams, and with the family is vital. The balance must nonetheless be achieved between individuals and agencies sharing information fully, so as to maximise provision, and risking breach of confidentiality. The European Standards on Confidentiality in Healthcare state that:

Service providers must establish and ensure the adoption of clear, publicly accessible, protocols for information sharing within teams, beyond teams and with outside organisations. Where it is planned to involve staff from other agencies this should first be discussed with the patient and/or their legal representative. The purpose of involving the other agency should be clarified along with the purpose of the contemplated information sharing. (McLelland 2006)

The use of processes and documentation that enable assessment, organisation and delivery of services to be provided effectively and efficiently requires services and individuals to share information. However, children, young people and their families should be made aware that individual professionals and services will share information, the reasons for this, and their rights related to this. Professionals also need to be clear on the purpose of information sharing. It's focus should be to facilitate the provision of a seamless service, with information shared only because of its relevance to the child, young person and their family and the support, treatment or care that they need or receive.

Education appears to provide some specific challenges in relation to services working together. Berry and Dawkins (2004) have identified a common feature of education for children with complex health needs being the failure of health and education authorities to work together at a local level to meet the needs of pupils. There can be confusion over whose responsibility it is to provide support for children who have medical needs whilst they are at school. The level of understanding that school staff have of a child's health needs and the support which they have in meeting these is also significant in determining whether the child is given the maximum possible opportunity to participate in education. As Chapter 2 identified, many children who have complex health needs miss school unnecessarily because there is no one present who can meet their health needs or because aspects of their condition are misunderstood. They may also be unnecessarily excluded from certain activities, or miss hours of education when this could be avoided if there was greater clarity regarding their healthcare needs and the management of these (Berry and Dawkins 2004).

Case study

Naz is 12. He has cerebral palsy, severe epilepsy, and is fed via a gastrostomy.

Naz enjoys school and the school he attends are excellent at developing his skills and abilities. However, they find his seizures hard to manage. Naz is always accompanied by a carer, but the school are concerned about what will happen if a school nurse is not on the premises and he has a seizure which is not self-limiting. They have therefore decided that if the school nurse is not present, he cannot attend.

Last year, the school nurse was off sick for two weeks. Naz missed two weeks of school because of this.

When services are provided in a way that divides provision between a range of providers and individuals, great efforts and co-ordination are required and for families to be effectively supported in a manner that meets their individual needs. Whilst individual practitioners may seek to work collaboratively, joint working is required at three levels to facilitate the provision of a truly joined up service: strategic planning agencies need to jointly plan provision; service commissioning needs to be collaborative and funding of service provision have the potential to be joined-up; and individuals who support the family on a day-to-day basis must work effectively together (Widdas et al. 2005; Boddy et al. 2006). Both the Department for Education and Skills and the Department of Health have an important role to play in encouraging pooled budgeting and joint service commissioning across agencies including health, education and social care (Boddy et al. 2006).

THE KEY WORKER

A vital part of successful multi agency and multiprofessional working is that the activities, decisions and services which will be provided by one individual or service are clearly and promptly communicated to other agencies and the child or young person and their family. In order to achieve this, having one named individual acting as the Key Worker who is the main point of advice, contact and co-ordination of services for the child or young person and their family has been identified as important (Department of Health 2004a, Boddy et al. 2006).

It seems logical that joined up assessment, planning and provision of support can only be truly effective where there is a clear and integrated channel of communication for all individuals. The role of the Key Worker therefore logically seems pivotal in the success of joined-up working and the provision of quality support, and a necessary investment. However, Kirk and Glendinning (2004) found that few families have a designated person who acts in such a role. In addition, where Key Workers do exist, Greco et al. (2006) found considerable variations in their views and understanding of their roles, and the amount of training and support which they receive.

Case study

Hope is 12. She has cerebral palsy, epilepsy, visual impairment and hearing difficulties. She is fed via a gastrostomy and requires assisted ventilation at night.

Hope has input from the homecare team from her local Primary Care Trust, the community children's nursing services, social services, her school, the local education authority, ophthalmic services and audiology services. She also has input from speech and language therapists while she is at school, a physiotherapist, occupational therapist and dietician. She sees a respiratory consultant, a gastroenterologist, a neurologist, an orthopaedic surgeon and a paediatrician. All these individuals and services discuss her needs with her and her mother, Constance. However, with so many people involved, Constance has always found it hard to make sure that everyone has the same goals, and understands the whole picture of what is happening with Hope.

Six months ago, Julia took on the role of Hope's Key Worker. Constance describes how this means that: 'I no longer have to co-ordinate everything. I used to spend literally hours every week trying to make sure that everyone had passed messages to each other. Now Julia does that. If I tell her that two people seem to be saying different things, she gets in touch with them, and she comes back to me and often we find they are aiming for the same thing, they just say it in different ways. Or she gets them to agree a plan they will both work from. She does the chasing for me. I don't have the phone calls to consultant's secretaries, and physio departments, and the school, asking them to talk to each other. You wouldn't believe how much my phone bill has gone down since she took over and how much more time I have to spend with Hope, being her Mum, not her secretary.'

ORGANISING CARE PACKAGES

Although home care is usually a cheaper option than hospital based care, supporting a child or young person who has complex health needs in their home requires substantial funding (Stalker et al. 2003). However, despite considerable financial investment in such services, there is evidence that these do not always provide the type of support that children and their families value (Noyes 2006b). A major factor in the quality of support provided is whether this places the child and their family centrally and treats them as people, both as individuals and as a family unit. Providing high-quality support requires the needs and priorities of the child and family, not the priorities or perceptions of service providers to be placed first. It also requires support to be provided in a way that will help the child or young person to do what is important for them and enable the family to achieve their potential as individuals and a family (Abbott et al. 2005).

The way in which the practicalities of provision of staff is managed is an important part of achieving a high-quality service. Continuity of the staff providing support is important for families and whether staff can fit in with the family, and form a good relationship with the whole family is also vital (Kirk and Glendinning 2004; Hewitt-Taylor 2007). However, this can be a challenge when services have to arrange provision for a range of families as the personalities, values, beliefs and attitudes of staff and families vary greatly and staff who work well with one family may not work well with another. Whilst matching staff and families closely is highly desirable, it can be very difficult for service providers to achieve this.

Recruiting staff can be difficult in any event and recruiting enough staff who match all the requirements of service providers and families can be almost impossible. Some organisations involve families in staff selection, but in other cases the number of families which a service caters for make this logistically impossible (Hewitt-Taylor 2007). One option is to have parent or family representatives on interview panels. This provides some user involvement, and input from those with a better insight into the perspectives of families than service providers may have. Nevertheless, given families' variations in preferences, personalities and priorities, it may come no closer to matching staff and families.

How families can have maximum choice in when, how and by whom support is provided is a vital consideration in quality provision. A challenge for service providers is to consider how best to maximise the quality of support for all families within real world constraints. A part of this is making explicit to all concerned at the outset each party's expectations, and limits of what can be provided, stating what will be their maximum choice within this, and then ensuring this is delivered. Although absolute choice over staff will not usually be available to families, as Chapters 4 and 5 describe, there may be cases where a particular staff member and family cannot work effectively together. Service providers should have in place strategies and mechanisms for dealing sensitively with such issues and families should be made aware not only of this potential, but of what will and will not be deemed reasonable expectations in this respect.

The vast majority of the day-to-day care of children who have complex health needs is carried out by staff who are not Registered Nurses, for example by Healthcare Support Workers. Kirk and Glendinning (2004) found that families are generally happy with this provided that the staff who provide them with support are familiar with the child, their needs and their treatment. What is more important to parents than level of qualification which an individual has is how far they see their child and family as individuals and people, and the way in which they work with, care for and about them (Kirk and Glendinning 2004; Hewitt-Taylor 2007).

Registered Nurses who lead teams composed mainly of Healthcare Support Workers who work alone in the family home must nonetheless be aware of how this affects their role and professional responsibilities. Delegation of responsibilities must still meet the Nursing and Midwifery Council (2004:8) requirement which states that:

> delegation must not compromise existing care but must be directed to meeting the needs and serving the interests of patients and clients.

Trained nurses who lead such teams:

remain accountable for the appropriateness of the delegation and for ensuring that the person who does the work is able to do it and that adequate supervision and support is provided.

This requires clarity over roles and lines and levels of responsibility, including the responsibilities that support workers have as employees, when they should refer to Registered Nurses or other individuals, the mechanisms by which this should be done, the role and responsibilities of families, where responsibilities overlap, and the ways in which concerns should be raised and addressed.

INDEPENDENT FUNDING OPTIONS

One option for families to enable them to gain greater control of their lives, the way in which support is provided, when, where and by whom is the use of Direct Payments (Department of Health 2007). Direct payments are payments for people who have been assessed as needing help from social services, and who want to arrange and pay for their own care and support services instead of receiving them directly from the local council.

Direct Payments can be made to adults, and to the parents or those with parental responsibility for disabled children (aged 0–17 years) and to 16- and 17-year-old disabled young people. Direct Payments must be spent on services which it has been agreed that Social Services will provide. The amount of a Direct Payment should cover the cost of obtaining a service of the same quality and quantity as social services would otherwise provide to meet the needs that a person has been assessed as having. The recipients of Direct Payments are obliged to keep an account of the money and its use (Department of Health 2007).

Persons with parental responsibility for a disabled child have a right to request an assessment of their needs in their capacity as carers, which may enable them to be awarded some financial assistance. The Carers and Disabled Children Act (HMSO 2000) also gives local councils the power to supply certain services directly to carers who have been assessed as needing them.

In healthcare, arrangements that enable funding for service provision to be supplied directly to individuals to enable them to organise their own support have not traditionally been possible. However, there have recently been inroads into exploring the possibility of developing a system similar to Direct Payments for healthcare provision (Alakeson 2007). There is some evidence from the USA to support this approach and its value in giving service users the option of more personalised support. Early evidence suggests that this improves service user satisfaction and outcomes, and tends to be of equal cost, or lesser cost, but are rarely more expensive than provision of services by NHS or Primary Care Trusts (Alakeson 2007).

Whilst managing their own support is appealing to many families, it can also increase their workload significantly. The estimate of the cost of the support that families need should include funding to provide them with assistance with day-to-day facilitation of the process of managing their support (Alakeson 2007). It is also recommended that if such an approach is adopted, mechanisms exist within it for families to be provided with assistance or guidance on issues such as employment law and financial management.

The development of this type of arrangement for support related to health needs may provide a very valuable and cost-effective option for many families and address the difficulties that large organisations face in recruiting staff who must be matched to a range of families. It may also, through the formation of such systems as Family Led Trusts commissioned via Primary Care Trusts facilitate a natural progression from families managing their child's care package to the young person managing their own package of care with appropriate support.

As with the intention of Direct Payments in social care, the development of options for families to receive funding to manage their own healthcare support must not preclude families who would prefer not to manage their own support continuing to use traditional service provision mechanisms.

SHORT-BREAK SERVICES

Where a child or young person has complex and continuing health needs, providing parents with short-break services so that they can have some time off from their role as carers is important (Neufeld et al. 2001; Olsen and Maslin-Prothero 2001; Department of Health 2004a; MacDonald and Callery 2004; Heaton et al. 2005). Yantzi et al. (2006) identify that there is a misconception that friends, families and neighbours can provide parents whose children have complex health needs with breaks from caring in the same way that they could with other children. The nature of some children's needs are such that family and friends are often unable to care for them, particularly for long periods of time, unless they have undergone specific additional training. They may not feel confident to take on such roles, and families may feel reluctant to allow them to take on such responsibility (Hewitt-Taylor 2007). This can mean that unless parents are provided with short-break services, some never have the opportunity to be away from their role as their child's carer. For many families, short-break services are essential to enable them to continue their role in caring for their child, and parents often use this time to sleep and combat the exhaustion that their child's care needs occasion (MacDonald and Callery 2004).

As well as the benefits for families, short-break services can be advantageous for children and young people (Department of Health 2004a). Where this gives them the opportunity to meet other children and young people, it can provide them with the chance to form friendships and be involved in social activities, new experiences and peer relationships which would not otherwise be available to them.

The key to high-quality short-break care provision is that it should be flexible and offer the child, young person and their family a choice about the type and location of services that they receive (Department of Health 2001a). Some children, young people and families prefer short-break care to be provided at home whilst others prefer to use an out of home facility (MacDonald and Callery 2004). For some parents their child being away from home for a short time allows them to engage with the outside world and to avoid having strangers in their home (MacDonald and Callery 2004). However, Heaton et al. (2005) also identify that families may prefer short-break care to be provided in their home, because the child or young person remains in a familiar environment, bulky equipment does not need transporting, and the staff who support them are familiar to and trusted by them. These last two points may be overcome out of the home when the carers who usually work with the family also provide their short-break care or if equipment can be replicated in other settings (Hewitt-Taylor 2007).

Despite the aim of providing choice for children, young people and their families in relation to short-break services, the reality is that funding and the availability of this type of care may limit the choices that families have. Short-break care provision is one of parents' most frequently reported unmet needs or problems (Department of Health 2004a, Kirk and Glendinning 2004). There are often waiting lists for short-break care, and children who have complex health needs and those with profound disabilities are more likely to have to wait for such services than others. The children and young people who have the greatest needs seem to have to wait the longest to have these met (Shared Care Network 2003). As the number of children and young people who have complex and continuing health needs increases, so too does the pressure on existing short-break provision.

A significant amount of short-break care provision is currently met by children's hospices, either by providing respite care at the hospice or via a home care team from the hospice. However, children's hospices are voluntary bodies, unevenly scattered throughout the country and often heavily subscribed to (Heaton et al. 2003). Many children's hospices have had to reduce the amount of short-break time which families have, because of the increasing demands on their services (Hewitt-Taylor 2007).

Families often need breaks during school holidays, and short-break care that is flexible and responsive to sudden changes in the family's circumstances (Department of Health 2004a). However, short-break services usually have to be planned in advance, and accessing provision at short notice, for example, if a parent becomes unwell is often very difficult (Olsen and Maslin-Prothero 2001; Hewitt-Taylor 2007).

Case study

Abigail is six. She has tracheomalacia and requires assisted ventilation at night. She also has severe epilepsy. Abigail has three siblings: Jordan aged 15, Eloise aged 10 and Dylan aged eight. The family have carers at night to supervise Abigail and one weekend in four short-break care at the local children's hospice. This means that during those weekends Abigail's parents can focus on what the other children want to do, without having to worry about whether Abigail can be taken to venues, whether she will need treatment during the day, and whether they will be home in time to set up her ventilator.

Because of the increased demands on services, their short-break care is being reduced to one weekend in eight. Abigail's mother, Hazel explains: 'For us, as a family, that means: I used to say to the others, "OK, every month one of you gets to choose what you want to do." So they chose, only four times a year, but they chose. Now it will be twice a year. Also, Abi actually likes it there. She has good friends there. Now she will see them less.'

SUMMARY

There are a range of ways in which children and young people who have complex and continuing health needs and their families can be provided with support. These include the provision of information, practical support and emotional support. The type of support that each family wants and how and when they would prefer this to be provided will vary. The constraints of resources will also affect what can be provided. However, within the constraints of the available resources, support should aim to provide what the family perceive will enable them to achieve the best possible quality of life, rather than what service providers think is needed or important. Short-break services are vital for many families, but require significant expansion and as much flexibility as possible. Service provision also needs to take into account contingency planning for situations where families need additional support at short notice.

In many cases families require input from a number of services, organisations and individuals. This creates a need for services and individuals to devise ways of working effectively together. Common assessment and planning strategies are important to optimise consistency of information gathering and giving and to avoid unnecessary repetition. Families having a Key Worker who acts as a central point of contact for them and all services and individuals involved in the provision of support is a vital part of providing services that are well co-ordinated and which lessen, rather than increase, parents' workloads.

The provision of staff to support families in their homes provides some specific challenges, but should aim to offer the maximum possible choice and flexibility to their needs. This will always need to be within realistic financial and practical constraints, but these and the limits within which negotiation can occur should be clear to families and service providers. For many families, the opportunity for provision of direct funding to enable them to purchase their own support across health and social care seems ideal. However, there should also be no requirement for parents to take this responsibility on, and those who take this route should be provided with the opportunity to be supported with the processes involved in the management of their child's support.

Chapter 11
Working with Children, Young People and Their Families

SEEING THE CHILD OR YOUNG PERSON FIRST

The number of children and young people who have what are described as complex and continuing health needs is increasing. Absolute clarity over how a child or young person is defined as having complex and continuing health needs is elusive and may even be unhelpful, by focusing on their health needs rather than on seeing them as a person. Whilst children and young people who are described in this way have a variety of health related needs, they should be seen first and foremost as children and young people, not identified or defined by their physical or medical needs. Identification of the impact that a child or young person's health needs has on them and their family, and how this can best be managed is clearly vital. However, the focus should be on providing support that facilitates as high as possible a quality of life for children, young people and their families, not assistance which simply meets their physical needs. Whilst technical competence and knowledge of a person's health related needs are essential, high-quality support requires staff to show respect for children and young people as individuals and as a part of their family. The support they require because of their health needs should be organsied and provided in a way that contributes to, rather than detracts from, enabling them to achieve what is important for them, and what they see as quality of life.

Whatever their medical or technical needs, children and young people who have complex health needs have the same rights as other children and young people, including the right to be involved in all the decisions that affect them. The influence that their perceptions, views and priorities are given will be affected by their age and level of understanding, but their understanding and ability to make choices should not be confused with their physical abilities or their ability to communicate verbally.

Communication is a vital part of every aspect of everyday life. Thus, if children and young people are not enabled to communicate, to develop their confidence in this and to see it as valuable, every aspect of their lives will be affected. If children and young people cannot communicate, or are not given the opportunity to do so, they will not be able to make choices, and to express their preferences. They will not be able to explain their basic likes and dislikes, what activities they would like to be involved in, and whether or not they are comfortable. Their relationships with their peers will be affected and they are unlikely to feel included or to achieve full inclusion in society.

Effective communication is essential if the child or young person's priorities, values and aspirations are to be central to the provision of support. This may be challenging where children and young people have difficulties in communicating verbally, or have sensory impairments such as hearing or sight loss. This requires staff to be adept in communicating, and be prepared to learn from children, young people, their families and other specialists about how to understand the child or young person's way of making their views known, and the best way to communicate with them. They may need to encourage others to take the time to listen to children and young people, and enabling children and young people to access advocacy services may also be beneficial.

Children and young people who have complex health needs have the same right to enjoy play activities and leisure pursuits as their peers. There are many practical challenges to achieving this, and many instances where the facilities which are provided do not cater for children and young people who have additional needs. However, service provision should aim to enable children and young people to enjoy as many opportunities to engage in play and leisure activities and to be with and a part of their peer group as possible.

Children and young people who have complex health needs have the right to education, and the support with which they are provided should again have the aim of facilitating this. Inclusion in education means a great deal more than a child or young person being enrolled in a mainstream school. It means children and young people being offered the same opportunities to achieve their potential that other children and young people have, and to engage in the full range of activities within school life. There needs to be liaison between health, social care and education providers so that the child or young person's physical needs can be catered for and so that they do not lose the opportunities that education offers through misunderstanding of their needs or how these can be met, or inclarity over which service has responsibility for meeting their needs whilst they are at school or college.

THE CHILD OR YOUNG PERSON AS A PART OF THEIR FAMILY

A child or young person having complex and continuing health needs has the potential to impact not only on themselves, and every aspect of their life, but on every aspect of their family's life. The support that is provided for children and young people should see them as a part of their family, and take into account how their needs and the provision for these may impact on all the members of the family, and on the child or young person's ability to be an active part of their family. Families are as unique as the individuals who make up the family unit, and supporting children, young people and their families effectively requires staff to have some insight into the way in which the family is structured, who is important to the child or young person, who should be and has the legal right to be involved in their lives, and in decision making with them.

Supporting a child or young person at home often centres on working very closely with their parents to facilitate their care and support needs. The relationship that is formed between staff and parents can be as vital as the one which staff have with the child or young person themselves. Whilst no assumptions should be made about what another person is feeling or values, having some insight into the experiences that parents may have had and continue to have as their child's mother or father can assist staff in providing sensitive support. This includes understanding some of the challenges that parents face day to day because of their child's needs and the provision for these; how their child's needs have affected their parents' expectations and lives; and how they feel that they and their child are valued and supported by professionals and society. It also involves recognising the distinction between what they feel for their child as a person, and their relationship with them, and the stress and frustrations which can occur because of the provision for their needs.

Working with children who have complex health needs and their families usually entails working with parents who are experts in their child and their needs. Working in the family home requires staff to respect the family as people, their values, priorities and home. It also requires them to respect and work with parents' childcare practices (except in cases where this would constitute harm to the child), to be able to learn from parents who are experts not only in their child's medical or technical care, but in them as people. Staff who work closely with families should aim to engage in a relationship of equal respect and mutual sharing for the benefit of the child or young person.

Although many parents whose children have complex health needs require assistance to enable their child to live at home, it is important to recognise that whilst they may need assistance with their child's care, this support is only required because of the extraordinary workload they have. Caring for a child who has complex and continuing health needs can be exhausting for parents. However, many of the stressors they experience come from the demands brought by their child's physical needs, the problems inherent in organising services and trying to overcome barriers which society places in their way, not the child themselves. The child is often a source of great reward and pleasure for their parents. The support provided should have as its aim enabling parents and families to enjoy the rewards, and pleasures which their child brings and the relationship which they have with them.

WORKING IN THE FAMILY HOME

Working with children and young people who have complex and continuing health needs and their families in their home can be very rewarding, but also presents staff and families with very specific challenges. Negotiating the roles that staff will take on and the relationship which they will have with the family is very different from the negotiation needed in most other settings. In addition, as staff often work with families over long periods of time, the fine tuning of the relationship is subject to almost constant informal negotiation. This applies not only to the relationship between staff and families but to the rules or accepted practices that apply to what is the family's home and staffs' workplace.

Staff who work closely with families in their homes have to negotiate the delicate balance between providing the family with support and becoming an unwelcome intrusion into their lives. They also have to be aware of and to be able to work with the fact that although families value the support they provide, in most cases they would ideally prefer to be able to care for their child alone. There are many factors that make it difficult for staff not to intrude on the privacy of families, but thinking about how these can be minimised and being aware of the range of ways in which their presence can be an intrusion may enable staff to reduce these. One of the essential skills of working with families in their home is to achieve the balance between concerned interest in the child's well-being and how this affects the family and over-involvement and emotional intrusion on the family. Despite being a vital skill, achieving this is possibly one of the greatest challenges of working with families in their homes.

One of the necessary considerations in the organisation and delivery of support in the family home is an acknowledgement that because of the human interactions that must occur, where personalities are such that an effective working relationship cannot be achieved, staff may need to stop working with a family simply on the grounds of unmatched personalities. This will obviously have to be within overall service constraints, but should be seen as an almost inevitable, if occasional, event, with no blame attached on either side in the majority of cases.

It is expedient, when working in the family home, for professionals and families to have some form of agreement regarding what each party can reasonably expect from the other. Although families' rights and privacy should be a prime concern for staff, staff also have the right to safety and well-being at work. Whilst there are some differences in interpretation of the Health and Safety at Work Act when the workplace is a private home, staff should not tolerate or be expected to tolerate known risks to their personal safety and well-being. Staff who work in the home setting have a responsibility to make their managers aware of any concerns they have regarding the safety of their workplace and mangers have a responsibility to act on these.

SUPPORTING YOUNG PEOPLE

An increasing number of children who have complex and continuing health needs are now living into adulthood and this means that there is a developing population of adolescents who have this type of health need. Although many of the principles that underpin providing effective support for children and their families apply equally to young people, there are some specific considerations for staff who work with adolescents who have complex and continuing health needs. Young people who have complex health needs may find the transition to independence much more difficult to achieve than their peers, because of their needs and the way in which these are provided for, but also because of the attitudes that society has towards them. Young people who have complex health needs may face many barriers to being enabled to become independent, to spending their leisure time with their peers, and to accessing further education and employment opportunities. The sexual needs of disabled people are generally poorly recognised and provided for and this is likely to be the same, if not more so, for young people who have complex health needs. These are all issues which those who support young people should take into account and the support provided should enable them to develop their maximum level of independence and to have the same opportunities as their peers.

Some of the challenges that young people who have complex health needs face will clearly be outside the influence of those providing their day-to-day support, however, the way in which support is organised and provided should have as a central tenet their need to have the same chances as other young people. This includes enabling young people to make their own choices, as other young people would, even where this may not be in line with what staff see as acceptable. Generally, unless protection of vulnerable people from harm by others is an issue, young people should not, on the grounds that they have complex health needs, be less permitted to make their own decisions about their lives and to take risks than other young people. Where young people are unused to making choices, or find it difficult to do so, an independent and supportive adult, such as an advocate, may be useful to enable them to learn how to make their own decisions, and to develop independence in expressing their choices and ensuring that these are acted on.

High-quality service provision for young people who have complex health needs includes an effective and person-centred transition to adult services. This usually requires advanced and diligent planning, and is usually best co-ordinated via a Key Worker or Lead Professional who can work closely with the young person to ensure that their voice is heard, listened to, and acted on in decisions affecting them.

DECISION MAKING AND FINITE RESOURCES

Although choice and control for children, young people and their families should be the mainstay of providing them with support, there is finite funding for what is increasingly an infinite demand for healthcare. This means that it will not always be possible to provide everything an individual or family needs or would like to enable them to avail themselves of all the opportunities which they could perhaps enjoy, and to fulfil all their hopes and aspirations. Whilst meeting the needs of individuals and families and placing centrally what they perceive as quality of life, the reality is that all of the needs which everyone has cannot be met by the funding available to the National Health Service. However, open and truthful dialogue should occur with children, young people and their families regarding the resources available to them, the choices they have, and the limits of these so that they can make decisions within what is available. A part of autonomous decision making is having access to full information, and a part of this is the reality that funding is not unlimited. Being truthful, which is an obligation for healthcare staff, includes giving children, young people and their families a truthful account of what can or cannot be provided, so that families can make informed choices and be aware of what provision they can expect.

For many children, young people and families, the provision of direct funding to enable them to purchase their own support across health and social care seems ideal, as it has the potential to offer them the optimum flexibility, choice and control in meeting their needs within the resources available. However, this also requires support and facilitation to be available to families who take on this responsibility, and there should also be no requirement for parents to take on the responsibility for managing their child's support if this option is developed.

Although the focus on decision making should be to enable children and their families to be autonomous in decision making, a clear distinction has to be made between autonomy and unsupported isolation. Respect for the autonomy of all human beings means that children, young people and their families should be supported and enabled to make their own decisions. This should nevertheless occur in a manner that conveys compassion, interest and supportive listening and which enables individuals and families to explore what is likely to be the best option for them. Children, young people and their families have to live with the outcomes of the decisions which they make. Whilst autonomy brings with it responsibility, the difficulties inherent in making decisions when outcomes are largely unknown should be acknowledged and children, young people and their parents enabled to discuss their concerns, fears and conflicting opinions without fear of judgement or obligation to accept the views of professionals. Professionals should aim to understand families' perspectives, and, whilst explaining their own knowledge, perspectives and values is an important part of any discussion, they should be clear that these are presented only in order to give individuals a full range of information from which to make decisions. This is a very different stance from attempting to coerce others, by whatever means, to accept their views.

Children, young people and their families are ultimately those who will know best what is important to them. This assumption, and respect for them, as individuals, as families, and for their homes should be the mainstay of providing community based support for children and young people who have complex and continuing health needs.

Appendix
Useful Resources

There are a number of support groups related to specific diseases, disorders or conditions which children, young people, their families and healthcare staff may find useful. Many of these are listed at:
http://www.surgerydoor.co.uk/sg/

A list of support groups and organisations can also be found at:
   http://www.direct.gov.uk/en/CaringForSomeone/CaringForADisabled Child/DG_10026501
   Other organisations or resources which children, young people, families or staff may find useful include the following.

ACE Centre
This centre provides a variety of services including in-depth individual assessments, information, and specialist training for parents and professionals on the use of technology for young people with physical and communication difficulties.
http://www.ace-centre.org.uk

Afasic (Unlocking Speech and Language)
A UK charity which represents children and young people who have communication impairments, works for their inclusion in society and supports their parents and carers.
http://www.afasic.org.uk

Changing Places
The Changing Places Consortium has launched a campaign on behalf of people who cannot use standard accessible toilets.
http://www.changing-places.org/

Contact a Family
A UK-wide charity providing support, advice and information for families with disabled children.
http://www.cafamily.org.uk/

Crossroads: Caring for Carers
An organisation that provides practical support for carers.
http://www.crossroads.org.uk

Carers Information
This site provides articles, documents, links and other resources to support informal carers.
http://www.carersinformation.org.uk/

Carers UK
An organisation that provides carers, those supporting them, and others with information about the benefits to which they are entitled.
http://www.carersuk.org

Family Fund
An organisation that champions an inclusive society where families with severely disabled children have choices and the opportunities to enjoy ordinary life.
http://www.familyfund.org.uk

ICAN
A charity that provides a combination of specialist therapy and education for children with the most severe and complex needs, and researches how to support these children most effectively.
http://www.ican.org.uk

KIDS
A national charity dedicated to helping children and young people with disabilities and special needs to develop their skills and abilities and to realise their potential.
http://www.kids-online.org.uk

Motability
A national charity that provides practical assistance to help disabled people to become mobile. This includes financial help and technical services.
http://www.motability.co.uk

Parents for Inclusion
A network of parents of disabled children and those who have special needs who work to promote inclusion in all areas of life, including education.
http://www.parentsforinclusion.org.

Shared Care Network
An organisation that promotes family based short breaks for disabled children in England, Wales and Northern Ireland.
http://www.sharedcarenetwork.org.uk/

Sibs
A charity for people who grow up with a brother or sister with special needs, disability, or chronic illness.
http://www.sibs.org.uk/

Skill
A national charity promoting opportunities for young people and adults with any kind of disability in post-16 education, training and employment across the UK.
http://www.skill.org.uk

Special Kids in the UK
A charity for families who have a child of any age with special needs.
http://www.specialkidsintheuk.org/

The Princess Royal Trust for Carers
This Trust provides information, advice and support for carers (including young carers).
http://www.carers.org/

UK Children on Long Term Ventilation
A website intended for the benefit of families and healthcare staff involved in supporting children and young people who require long-term assisted ventilation.
http://www.longtermventilation.nhs.uk/

Whizz-Kidz

Provides children who have mobility problems with customised wheelchairs, tricycles and other specialised mobility equipment, as well as providing training and advice.
http://www.whizz-kidz.org.uk

Young Carers Net

Provides information and support for young carers.
http://www.youngcarers.net

References

Abbott D Howarth J (2007) Still off limits? Staff views on supporting gay, lesbian and bisexual people with learning disabilities to develop sexual and intimate relationships. *Journal of Applied Research in Intellectual Disabilities*, 20(2), 116–126.

Abbott D Watson D Townsley R (2005) The proof of the pudding: what difference does multi-agency working make to families with disabled children with complex healthcare needs? *Child and Family Social Work*, 10(3), 229–238.

Alakeson V (2007) The Case for Extending Direct Payments into the NHS - Evidence from the USA. Office of the Assistant Secretary for Planning and Evaluation Department of Health and Human Services, Washington DC.

Anderson P Kitchin R (2000) Disability, space and sexuality: access to family planning services. *Social Sciences and Medicine*, 51(8), 1163–1173.

Appierto L Cori M Binnchi R Onofri A Catena S Ferrari M Villani A (2002) Home care for chronic respiratory failure in children: 15 years experience. *Paediatric Anaesthesia*, May 12(4), 345–350.

Atwal A Caldwell K (2006) Nurses' perceptions of multidisciplinary team work in acute healthcare. *International Journal of Nursing Practice*, 12(6), 359–365.

Audit Commission (1993) *Children First: a study of hospital services*. HMSO, London.

Balling K McCubbin M (2001) Hospitalized children with chronic illness: parental caregiving needs and valuing parental expertise. *Journal of Pediatric Nursing*, 16(2), 110–119.

Barr O Millar R (2003) Parents of children with intellectual disabilities: their expectations and experience of genetic counselling. *Journal of Applied Research in Intellectual Disabilities*, 16(3), 189–204.

Bartlow B (2006) What, me grieve? Grieving and bereavement in daily dialysis practice. *Haemodialysis*, 10(2), S46–S50.

Beauchamp TL Childress JF (2001) *Principles of Biomedical Ethics*. Oxford University Press, Oxford.

Beresford B (2004) On the road to nowhere? Young disabled people and transition. *Child Care, Health and Development*, 30(6), 581–587.

Bernard C (1999) Child sexual abuse and the black disabled child. *Disability and Society*, 14(3), 325–340.

Berry T Dawkins B (2004) *Don't Count Me Out*. MENCAP, London.

Better Health (2001) Peer Pressure Factsheet. Better Health Channel. Victoria. Australia. http://www.disability.vic.gov.au/bhcv2/bhcpdf.nsf/ByPDF/Peer_pressure/$File/ Peer_pressure pdf accessed 31 August 2007.

Boddy J Potts P Stratham J (2006) *Models of Good Practice in Joined-up Assessment: working for children with 'significant and complex needs'*. Department for Education and Skills, London.

Boosfeld B O'Toole M (2000) Technology dependent children: from hospital to home. *Paediatric Nursing*, 12(6), 20–22.

Bradshaw J (1998) Assessing and intervening in the communication environment. *British Journal of Learning Disabilities* 26(1), 62–65.

Brazier M (2006) *Critical Care Decisions in Fetal and Neonatal Medicine: ethical issues*. Nuffield Council for Bioethics, London.

Breakey WJ (1997) Body image: the inner mirror. *Journal of Prosthetics and Orthotics*, 9(3), 107–112.

Brett J (2004) The journey to accepting support: how parenst of profoundly disabled children experience support in their lives. *Paediatric Nursing*, 16(8), 14–18.

Bridges J Hanson R Little M Flannigan AC Fairley M Haywood L (2001) Ethical relationships in paediatric emergency medicine: moving beyond the dyad. *Emergency Medicine*, 13(3), 344–350.

Bu X Jezewski MA (2006) Developing a mid-range theory of patient advocacy through concept analysis. *Journal of Advanced Nursing*, 57(1), 101–110.

Buelow JM McNelis A Shore CP Austin JK (2006) Stressors of parents of children with epilepsy and intellectual disability. *Journal of Neurosciences Nursing*, 38(3), 147–154, 176.

Burchardt T (2005) *The Education and Employment of Disabled Young People: frustrated ambition*. The Policy Press and Joseph Rowntree Foundation, Bristol.

Cambridge P (1999) The first hit: a case study of physical abuse of people with learning disabilities and challenging behaviour in a residential service. *Disability and Society*, 14(3), 285–306.

Canter R (2001) Patients and medical power. *British Medical Journal*, 323(7310), 414.

Carnevale FA Alexander E Davis M Renick J Troini R (2006) Daily living with distress and enrichment: the moral experience of families with ventilator-assisted children at home. *Pediatrics*, 117(1), 48–60.

Cavet J Sloper P (2004) Participation of disabled children in individual decisions about their lives and in public decisions about service development. *Children and Society* 18(4), 278–290.

Christensen M Hewitt-Taylor J (2006) Empowerment in nusring: paternalism or maternalism? *British Journal of Nursing*, 15(13), 695–699.

Christie D Viner R (2005) Adolescent development. *British Medical Journal*, 330(7486), 301–304.

Commission of Child Health Services (1976) *Fit for the Future* (The Court Report). HMSO, London.

Condliffe C (2006) Caring for children with complex health needs. *Journal of Community Nursing*, 20(6), 4–14.

Contact a Family (2004a) *Flexible Enough*? Contact a Family, London.

Contact a Family (2004b) *Relationships and Caring for a Disabled Child*. Contact a Family, London.

Contact a Family (2005) *Grandparents*. Contact a Family, London.

Contact a Family (2007) *Siblings. Information for families*. Contact a Family, London.

Corden A Sloper P Sainsbury R (2002) Financial effects for families after the death of a disabled or chronically ill child: a neglected dimension of bereavement. *Child Care, Health and Development*, 28(3), 199–204.

Cormack M A (2007) Parental responsibility: a legal perspective. *Journal of Children's and Young People's Nursing*, 1(4), 194.

Council of Europe (1950) *European Convention on Human Rights. Convention for the Protection of Human Rights and Fundamental Freedoms as amended by protocol no. 11*. Council of Europe, Rome.

Coulter A (1999) Paternalism or partnership? *British Medical Journal*, 319(7212), 719–720.

Coyle J (1999) Exploring the meaning of dissatisfaction with healthcare: the importance of personal identity threat. *Sociology of Health and Illness*, 21(1), 95–123.

Craft A (2004) Children with complex healthcare needs – supporting the child and family in the community. *Child Care, Health and Development*, 30(3), 193–194.

Da Silva CH Cunha RL Tonaco RB Cunha TM Diniz AC Domingos GG Silva JD Santos MV Antoun MG de Paula RL (2003) Not telling the truth in the patient-physician relationship. *Bioethics*, 17(5–6), 417–424.

Davies R (2004) New understandings of parental grief: literature review. *Journal of Advanced Nursing*, 46(5), 506–513.

Davis S Hall D (2005) 'Contact a family' professionals and parents in partnership. *Archives of Diseases in Childhood*, 90(10), 1053–1057.

Dearden C Becker S (2004) *Young Carers in the UK*. Carers UK and the Children's Society, London.

deCinque N Monterosso L Dadd G Sidhu R MacPherson R Aoun S (2006) Bereavement support for families following the death of a child from cancer: experience of bereaved parents. *Journal of Psychosocial Oncology*, 24(2), 65–83.

Department for Education and Skills (2006a) *The Common Assessment Framework for Children & Young People: Practitioners' Guide*. DfES, Nottingham.

Department for Education and Skills (2006b) *Working Together to Safeguard Children: a guide to interagency working to safeguard and promote the welfare of children*. HMSO, London.

Department for Education and Skills and Department of Health (2006) *Transition: getting it right for young people*. DoH, London.

Department of Health (1990) *The NHS and Community Care Act*. HMSO, London.

Department of Health (1998) *The National Service Framework for Paediatric Intensive Care*. DoH, Lonodn.

Department of Health (2000a) *The NHS Plan: A Plan for Investment; a Plan for Reform*. The Stationary Office, London.

Department of Health (2000b) *Framework for the Assessment of Children in Need and their Families*. The Stationary Office, London.

Department of Health (2001a) *Valuing People: a new strategy for learning disability for the 21st century*. HSMO, London.

Department of Health (2001b) *The Expert Patient*. DoH, London.

Department of Health (2004a) *The National Service Framework for Children, Young People and Maternity Services: disabled children and young people and those with complex health needs*. DoH, London.

Department of Health (2004b) *The Children Act*. HMSO, London.

Department of Health (2006) *Our Health, Our Care, Our Say: a new direction for community services*. DoH, London.

Department of Health (2007) Direct Payments: an introduction. http://www.dh. gov.uk/en/Policyandguidance/Organisationpolicy/Financeandplanning/ Directpayments/DH_4062246 accessed 24 August 2007.

Dimond B (1999) Legal issues arising in community nursing 1: health and safety. *British Journal of Community Nursing*, 4(9), 481–483.

Dimond B (2000) Legal issues arising in community nursing number 9: confidentiality. *British Journal of Community Nursing*, 5(8), 401–403.

Dimond B (2005) Legal aspects of community care of the sick child. In Sidey A Widdas D (Eds) *Textbook of Community Children's Nursing*, second edition, pp. 137–147. Elsevier, London.

Dodd LW (2004) Supporting the siblings of young children with disabilities. *British Journal of Special Education*, 31(1), 41–49.

Donaldson L (2003) Expert patients usher in a new era of opportunity for the NHS. *British Medical Journal*, 326(7402), 1279–1280.

Donovan M Vanleit B Crowe TK Keefe E (2005) Occupational goals of mothers of children with disabilities. *American Journal of Occupational Therapy*, 59(3), 249–261.

Draper H, Sorrell T (2002) Patients' responsibilities in medical ethics. *Bioethics*, 16(4), 335–352.

Dyer C (2004) Hospital breached boy's human rights by treating him against his mother's wishes. *British Medical Journal*, 328(7441), 661.

Dyregrov A (2002) *Grief in Children*. Jessica Kingsley, London.

Eakes GG Burke ML Hainsworth MA (1998) Middle-range theory of chronic sorrow. *Journal of Nursing Scholarship*, 30(2), 179–184.

Earle S (1999) facilitated sex and the concept of sexual need: disabled students and their personal assistants. *Disability and Society*, 14(3), 309–323.

Earle S (2001) Disability, facilitated sex and the role of the nurse. *Journal of Advanced Nursing*, 36(3), 433–444.

Edgar J Morton NS Pace NA (2001) Review of ethics in paediatric anaesthesia: intensive care issues. *Paediatric Anaesthesia*, 11(5), 597–601.

Edwards SD (1996) *Nursing Ethics: a principles based approach*. McMillan, Basingstoke.

Elston S (2003) *Assessment of Children with Life-limiting Conditions and their Families: A Guide to effective care planning*. Association for Children's Palliative Care, Bristol.

Encyclopaedia Britannica (2006) accessed via Britannica Online, http://www.britannica. com/ accessed 22 August 2007.

English D (2005) Moral obligations of patients: A clinical view. *Journal of Medicine and Philosophy*, 30(2), 139–152.

Farasat H Hewitt-Taylor J (2007) Learning to support children with complex and continuing health needs and their families. *Journal of Specialists in Pediatric Nursing*, 12(2), 72–83.

Farnalls SL, Rennick J (2003) Parents' caregiving approaches: facing a new treatment alternative in severe intractable childhood epilepsy. *Seizure*, 12(1), 1–10.

Feldstein SW Miller WR (2006) Substance use and risk taking amongst adolescents. *Journal of Mental Health*, 15(6), 633–643.

Fisher K Goodley D (2007) The linear medical model of disability: mothers of disabled babies resist with counter-narratives. *Sociology of Health & Illness*, 29(1), 66–81.

Fletcher L Buka P (1999) *A Legal Framework for Caring*. Palgrave, Basingstoke.

Freire P (1970) *Pedagogy of the Oppressed*. Penguin, London.

Gadow S (1989) Clinocal subjectivity:advocacy with silent patients. Nursing Clinics of North America, 24(2), 535–541.

Gage JD Everett KD Bullock L (2006) Integrative review of parenting in nursing research. *Journal of Nursing Scholarship*, 38(1), 56–62.

Gallant MH, Beaulieu MC, Carnevale FA (2002) Partnership: an analysis of the concept within the nurse-client relationship. *Journal of Advanced Nursing*, 40(2), 149–157.

George L (2005) Lack of preparedness: experiences of first-time mothers. American Journal of Maternal Child Nursing, 30(4), 251–255.

Gillick vs *West Norfolk and Wisbeach Health Authority* (1986) Appeal Cases 112–207.

Gilroy C Johnson P (2004) Listening to the language of children's grief. *Groupwork*, 14(3), 91–111.

Glendinning C Kirk S (2000) High tech care: high skilled parents. *Paediatric Nursing*, 12(6), 25–27.

Godfrey J (1999) Empowerment through sexuality. In Wilkinson G and Miers M (Eds) *Power and Nursing Practice*, pp. 172–186. Macmillan, London.

Goodyear-Smith F Buetow S (2001) Power issues in the doctor-patient relationship. *Health Care Analysis*, 9(4), 449–462.

Grace PJ (2001) Professional advocacy: widening the scope of accountability. *Nursing Philosophy*, 2(2), 151–162.

Greco V Sloper P (2004) Care coordination and key worker schemes for disabled children: results of a UK wide survey. *Child: Care, Health and Development*, 30(1), 13–20.

Greco V Sloper P Webb R Beecham J (2006) Key worker services for disabled children: the views of staff. *Health and Social Care in the Community*, 14(6), 445–452.

Green SE (2001) Grandma's hands: parental perceptions of the importance of grandparents as secondary caregivers in families of children with disabilities. *International Journal of Ageing and Human Development*, 53(1), 11–33.

Green SE (2002) Mothering Amanda: musings on the experience of raising a child with cerebral palsy. *Journal of Loss and Trauma*, 7(1), 21–34.

Green SE (2007) We're tired, not sad: benefits and burdens of mothering a child with disability. *Social Science and Medicine*, 64(1), 150–163.

Griffith R Stevens M (2004) Legal requirements for safe handling in community care. *British Journal of Community Nursing*, 9(5), 211–215.

Hall EO (2004) A double concern: grandmothers' experiences when a small grandchild is critically ill. *Journal of Pediatric Nursing*, 19(1), 61–69.

Hazel R (2006) The psychosocial impact on parents of tube feeding their child. *Paediatric Nursing*, 18(4), 19–22.

Heaton J Noyes J Sloper P Shah R (2003) *Technology and Time: home care regimes and technology – dependent children*. ESRC/MRC Innovative Health Technology research programme. SPRU University of York, York.

Heaton J Noyes J Sloper P Shah R (2005) Families' experiences of caring for technology dependent children: a temporal perspective. *Health and Social Care in the Community*, 13(5), 441–450.

Her Majesty's Stationery Office (1995) *The Disability Discrimination Act*. HMSO, London.

Her Majesty's Stationery Office (1998) *The Human Rights Act*. HMSO, London.

Her Majesty's Stationery Office (2000) *Carers and Disabled Children's Act*. HMSO, London.

Her Majesty's Stationery Office (2001) *The Special Educational Needs and Disability Act*. HMSO, London.

Her Majesty's Stationery Office (2005) *The Disability Discrimination Act*. HMSO, London.

Hewison A (1995) Nurses' power in interactions with patients. *Journal of Advanced Nursing*, 21(1), 75–82.

Hewitt J (2002) A critical review of the arguments debating the roles of the nurse advocate. *Journal of Advanced Nursing*, 37(5), 439–445.

Hewitt-Taylor J (2006) *Clinical Guidelines and Care Protocols*. Wiley, Chichester.

Hewitt-Taylor J (2007) *Children with Complex and Continuing Health Needs*. Jessica Kingsley, London.

Joffe S Manocchia M Weeks JC Cleary PD (2003) What do patients value in their hospital care? An empirical perspective on autonomy centered bioethics. *Journal of Medical Ethics*, 29(2), 103–108.

Johnson G (2006) Confidentiality and standards of care. *Midwives*, 9(12), 486–487.

Judson L (2004) Protective care: mothering a child dependent on parenteral nutrition. *Journal of Family Nursing*, 10(1), 93–120.

Kaplan C (2002) Children and the law: The place of health professionals. *Child and Adolescent Mental Health*, 7(4), 181–188.

Kearney P Griffin T (2001) Between joy and sorrow: being a parent of a child with developmental disability. *Journal of Advanced Nursing*, 34(5), 582–592.

Kelly P Uddin S (2005) Cultural issues in community children's nursing. In Sidey A Widdas D (Eds), *Textbook of Community Children's Nursing*, second edition, pp. 161–169. Elsevier, London.

Kennedy I (2003) Patients are experts in their own field. *British Medical Journal*, 326 (7402), 1276–1277.

Kerr SM McIntosh JB (2000) Coping when a child has a disability: exploring the impact of parent to parent support. *Child: Care, Health and Development*, 26(4), 309–322.

Kirk S (2001) Negotiating lay and professional roles in the care of children with complex healthcare needs. *Journal of Advanced Nursing*, 34(5), 593–602.

Kirk S Glendinning C (2004) Developing services to support parents caring for a technology dependent child at home. *Child: Care Health and Development*, 30(3), 209–218.

Kirk S Glendinning C Callery P (2005) Parent or nurse? the experience of being the parent of a technology dependent child. *Journal of Advanced Nursing*, 51(5), 456–464.

Kirklin D (2007) Truth telling, autonomy and the role of metaphor. *Journal of Medical Ethics*, 33(1), 11–14.

Koh A (1999) Non judgemental care as a professional obligation. *Nursing Standard*, 13(37), 38–41.

Krueger G (2006) Meaning making in the aftermatch of sudden infant death syndrome. *Nursing Inquiry*, 13(3), 163–171.

Kübler Ross E (1997) *On Death and Dying*. Touchstone, New York.

Landsman GH (1998) reconstructing motherhood in the age of 'perfect babies' mothers of infants and toddlers with disabilities. *Signs*, 24(1), 69–99.

Landsman G (2005) Mothers and models of disability. *Journal of Medical Humanities* 26(2/3), 121–139.

Lassetter JH Mandleco BL Roper SO (2007) Family photographs: expressions of parents raising children with disabilities. *Qualitative Health Research*, 17(4),456–567.

Lenton R (2006) Reining in autonomy? *Journal of the Royal College of Physicians of Edinburgh*, 36(2), .123

Leonardi M Bickenbach J Ustun TB Kostanjsek N Chatterji S (2006) The definition of disability: what is in a name? *The Lancet*, 368(9543), 1219–1221.

Levine C (2005) Acceptance, avoidance, and ambiguity: conflicting social values about childhood disability. *Kennedy Institute of Ethics Journal*, 15(4), 371–383.

Lowden J (2002) Children's rights: a decade of dispute. *Journal of Advanced Nursing*, 37(1), 100–107.

MacDonald H (2007) Relational ethics and advocacy in nursing: literature review. *Journal of Advanced Nursing*, 57(2), 119–126.

MacDonald H Callery P (2004) Different meanings of respite: a study of parents, nurses and social workers caring for children with complex needs. *Child: Care, Health and Development*, 30(3), 279–288.

Magnusson A Severinsson E Lutzen (2002) Nurses' views on situations related to privacy in providing home care for persons with long-term mental illness: an exploratory study. *Issues in Mental Health Nursing*, 23(1), 61–75.

Malin N Teasdale K (1991) Caring versus empowerment: considerations for nursing practice. *Journal of Advanced Nursing*, 16(6), 657–662.

Mallik M (1998) Advocacy in Nursing: perceptions and attitudes of the nursing elite in the United Kingdom. *Journal of Advanced Nursing*, 28(5), 1001–1011.

Mandana V (2007) The impact of health communication on health related decision making. *Health Education*, 107(1), 27–41.

McCann E (2000) The expression of sexuality in people with psychosis: breaking the taboos. *Journal of Advanced Nursing*, 32(1), 132–138.

McClure L (2005) Young carers and community children's nursing. In Sidey A Widdas D (Eds) *Textbook of Community Children's Nursing*, second edition, pp. 289–297. Elsevier, London.

McConkey R Smyth M (2003) Parental perceptions of risks with older teenagers who have severe learning difficulties contrasted with the young people's views and experiences. *Children and Society*, 17(1), 18–31.

McCourt C (2006) Becoming a parent. In Page LA McCandlish R (Eds) *The New Midwifery: Science and Sensitivity in Practice*, second edition, pp. 49–71. Churchill Livingstone, London.

McGrath P Holewa H McGrath Z (2006) Nursing advocacy in an Australian multidisciplinary context: findings on medico-centrism *Scandinavian Journal of Caring Sciences*, 20(4), 394–402.

McLelland R (2006) *European Standards on Confidentiality and Privacy in Healthcare*. Queen's University, Belfast, Belfast.

Meehan DR (2005) Mothering a 3- to 6-year-old child with hemiparesis. *Journal of Neurosciences Nursing*, 37(5), 265–271.

Menahem S Grimwade J (2003) Pregnancy termination following prenatal diagnosis of serious heart disease in the fetus. *Early Human Development*, 73(1), 71–78.

Millar S Aitken S (2005) *FE and Complex Needs. Views of children and young people.* Communication Aids for Language and Learning Centre, University of Edinburgh, Edinburgh.

Mitchell GJ, Bournes DA (2000) Nurse as patients advocate? In search of straight thinking. *Nursing Science Quarterly*, 13(3), 204–209.

Mok YS (2005) Respect based toleration. *Nursing Philosophy*, 6(4), 274–277.

Moser A Houtepen R Widdershoven G (2007) Patient autonomy in nurse led shared care: a review of theoretical and empirical literature. *Journal of Advanced Nursing*, 57(4), 357–365.

Mulligan S (2003) *Occupational Therapy Evaluation for Children: A pocket guide*. Lippincott Williams & Wilkins, Baltimore, MD.

Murray JS (2000) Understanding sibling adaptation to childhood cancer. *Issues in Comprehensive Paediatric Nursing*, 23(1), 39–47.

National Autistic Society (2007) Advocacy and Autism. http://www.nas.org.uk/nas/jsp/polopoly.jsp?d=296&a=10325 accessed 5 August 2007.

National Institute for Health and Clinical Excellence (2005) *A Guide to NICE*. NICE, London.

Nessa N (2004) *The Health of Children and Young People: Disability*. Office for National Statistics, London.

Neufeld SM Query B Drummond JE (2001) Respite care users who have children with chronic conditions: are they getting a break? *Journal of Pediatric Nursing*, 16(4), 234–244.

Noyes J (2006a) Health and quality of life of ventilator-dependent children. *Journal of Advanced Nursing*, 56(4), 392–403.

Noyes J (2006b) The KEY to success: managing children's complex packages of community support. *Archives of Diseases in Childhood: Education and Practice*, 91(4), ep106–ep110.

Noyes J Godfrey C Beecham J (2006) Resource use and service costs for ventilator-dependent children and young people in the UK. *Health and Social Care in the Community*, 14(6), 508–522.

Nursing and Midwifery Council (2002) *Practitioner-client Relationships and the Prevention of Abuse*. NMC, London.

Nursing and Midwifery Council (2004) *The NMC Code of Professional Conduct; standards for conduct, performance and ethics.* NMC, London.

Nuutila L Salantera S (2005) Children with long term illness: parents' experiences of care. *Journal of Pediatric Nursing,* 21(2), 153–160.

Nyatanga L Dann KL (2002) Empowerment in Nursing: the role of philosophical and psychological factors. Nursing Philosophy, 3(3), 234–239.

Nye RA (1999) *Sexuality.* Oxford University Press, Oxford.

O'Brien ME Wegner CB (2002) Rearing the child who is technology dependent: perceptions of parents and home care nurses. *Journal of Specialist Pediatric Nursing,* 7(1), 7–15.

Office of the United Nations High Commissioner for Human Rights (1989) *The United Nations Convention on the Rights of the Child.* Office of the United Nations High Commissioner for Human Rights, Geneva.

Ofsted (2004) Special education needs and disability: towards inclusive schools. HMI 2276. Ofsted. www.ofsted.gov.uk accessed 4 February 2007.

Olsen R Maslin-Prothero P (2001) Dilemmas in the provision of own-home respite support for parents of young children with complex healthcare needs: evidence from an evaluation. *Journal of Advanced Nursing,* 34(5), 603–610.

Olsen DP Dixon JK Grey M Deshefy-Longhi T Demarest JC (2005) Privacy Concerns of Patients and Nurse Practitioners in Primary Care. *Journal Of The American Academy Of Nurse Practitioners* 17(12), 527–534.

Orfali K Gordon E (2004) Autonomy gone awry: a cross-cultural study of parents' experiences in neonatal intensive care units. *Theoretical Medicine and Bioethics,* 25(4), 329–365.

Paediatric Intensive Care Society (2002) *Standards for Bereavement Care.* Paediatric Intensive Care Society, Sheffield.

Parkes CM, Markus A (Eds) (1998) *Coping with Loss: helping patients and their families.* BMJ Books, London.

Parekh SA (2006) Child consent and the law: an insight and discussion into the law relating to consent and competence. *Child Health, Care and Development,* 33(1), 78–82.

Parker G Bhakta P Lovett C Olsen R Paisley S Turner D (2006) Paediatric home care: a systematic reviews of randomized trails on costs and effectiveness. *Journal of Health Service Research Policy,* 11(2), 110–119.

Phoenix A Wollett A Lloyd E (1991) *Motherhood: meaning, practices and ideologies.* Sage, London.

Pierce D Marshall A (2004) Maternal management of home space and time to facilitate infant/toddlers play and development. In Esdaile SA Olson JA (Eds) *Mothering Occupations: Challenge, Agency and Participation,* pp. 73–94. FA Davis, Philadelphia, PA.

Platt H (1959) *The Welfare of Children in Hospital* (report of the committee). Ministry of Health commissioned report. Central Health Services, London.

Poses RM (2003) A cautionary tale: the dysfunction of American healthcare. *European Journal of Internal Medicine,* 14(2), 123–130.

Potgieter CA Gadija K (2005) Sexual self-esteem and body image of South African spinal cord injured adolescents. *Sexuality and Disability,* 23(1), 1–20.

Redmond B Richardson V (2003) Just getting on with it. exploring the service needs of mothers who car for young children with severe/profound and life threatening intellectual disability. *Journal of Applied Research in Intellectual Disabilities*, 16(4), 205–218.

Regnard C Reynolds J Watson B Matthews D Gibson L Clarke C (2007) Understanding distress in people with severe communication difficulties: developing and assessing the Disability Distress Assessment Tool (DisDAT). *Journal of Intellectual Disability Research*, 51(4), 277–292.

Rehm RS Bradley JF (2005) Normalization in families raising a child who is medically fragile/technology dependent and developmentally delayed. *Qualitative Health Research*, 15(6), 807–820.

Reyna VF Farley F (2006) Risk and rationality in adolescent decision making: implications for theory, practice, and public policy. *Psychological Science in the Public Interest*, 7(1), 1–44.

Riesz E (2004) Loss and transitions: A 30-year perspective on life with a child who has Down Syndrome. *Journal of Loss and Trauma*, 9(4), 371–382.

Riley M (2003) Facilitating children's grief. *Journal of School Nursing*, 19(4), 212–218.

Ronayne S (2001) Nurse: patient partnerships in hospital care. *Journal of Clinical Nursing*, 10(5), 591–592.

Rosenblatt PC (2000) *Parent Grief: narratives of loss and relationship*. Brunner-Mazl, Philadelphia, PA.

Rowse V (2007) Consent in severely disabled children: informed or an infringement of their human rights. *Journal of Child Healthcare*, 11(1), 70–77.

Royal College of Nursing (2003) *Defining Nursing*. Royal College of Nursing, London.

Russell P (2003) Access and Achievement or Social Exclusion? Are the Government's Policies Working for Disabled Children and Their Families? *Children and Society*, 17(3), 215–225.

Sakellariou D Algado SS (2006) Sexuality and disability: a case of occupational injustice. *British Journal of Occupational Therapy*, 69(2), 69–76.

Saldinger A Cain A Kalter N lohnes K (1999) Anticipating parental death in families with children. *American Journal of Orthopsychiatry*, 69(1), 39–47.

Salvage J (1990) The theory and practice of the 'new nursing'. *Nursing Times*, 86(4), 42–45.

Samwell B (2005) Nursing the family and supporting the nurse. In Sidey A Widdas D (Eds) *Textbook of Community Children's Nursing*, second edition, pp. 129–136. Elsevier, London.

Sanders R (2004) *Sibling Relationships*. Palgrave, Basingstoke.

Sant Angelo D (2000) Learning disability community nursing. Addressing emotional and sexual health needs. In Astor R Jeffries K (Eds) *Positive Initiatives for People with Learning Difficulties: Promoting Healthy Lifestyles*, pp. 52–68. MacMillan Press, Basingstoke.

Schalock RL Brown L Brown R Cummins RA Felce D Matikka L Keith KD Parmenter T (2002) Conceptualization, measurement and application of quality of life for people with intellectual disabilities: report of an international panel of experts. *Mental Retardation*, 40(6), 457–470.

Schifman LG Kanuk L (1996) *Consumer Behaviour*, sixth edition. Prentice Hall International, Englewood Cliffs, NJ.

Scorgie K Sobsey D (2000) Transformational outcomes associated with parenting children who have disabilities. *Mental Retardation*, 38(3), 195–206.

Scornaienchi JM (2003) Chronic sorrow: one mother's experience with two children with lissencephaly. *Journal of Paediatric Healthcare*, 17(6), 290–294.

Serwint J (2004) One method of coping: resident debriefing after the death of a patient. *Journal of Pediatrics*, 145(2), 229–234.

Seymour W (1998) *Remaking the Body. Rehabilitation and Change*. Routledge, London.

Shakespeare T (1999) The sexual politics of disabled masculinity. *Sexuality and Disability*, 17(1), 53–64.

Shared Care Network (2003) Too disabled to care? Shared Care Network, http://www.sharedcarenetwork.org.uk accessed 5 February 2007.

Sharland E (2006) Young People, Risk Taking and Risk Making: Some Thoughts for Social Work. Forum Qualitative Sozialforschung / Forum: Qualitative Social Research 7(1), Art. 23. Available at: http://www.qualitativeresearch.net/fqs-texte/1-06/06-1-23-e.htm, accessed 29 August 2007.

Sharpe D Rossiter L (2002) Siblings of children with a chronic illness: A meta-analysis. *Journal of Pediatric Psychology*, 27(8), 699–710.

Shenkman B Wegener D (2000) *Children with Special Healthcare Needs in the Healthy Kids Program*. Report to the Healthy Kids Corporation, 21 August 2000. Florida Healthy Kids Corporation, Tallahassee, FL.

Shier H (2001) Pathways to participation: opening opportunities and obligations. *Children and Society*, 15(2), 107–117.

Shribman S (2007) *Making it Better: for children and young people*. Department of Health, London.

Skar L (2002) Disabled children's perceptions of technical aids, assistance and peers in play situations. *Scandinavian Journal of Caring Sciences*, 16(1), 27–33.

Soanes C Stevenson A (2005) *Oxford Dictionary of English*. Oxford University Press, Oxford.

Soanes C Waite M Hawker S (2001) *Oxford Dictionary and Thesaurus*. Oxford University Press, Oxford.

Stalker K Carpenter J Phillips R Connors C MacDonald C Eyre J Noyes J Chaplin S Place M (2003) *Care and Treatment? Supporting children with complex needs in healthcare settings*. Pavilion Publishing, Brighton.

Steinberg L (2007) Risk taking in adolescence. New perspectives form brain and behavioural science. *Current Directions in Psychological Science*, 16(2), 55–59.

Stevens E (2006) *Definition Agreed By The Complex Needs Group*. Information Services, National Health Services Scotland, Edinburgh.

Stipek D Recchia S McClintic S (1992) Self-evaluation in young children. *Monographs of the Society for Research in Child Development*, 57(1), 1–98.

Strandmark MK (2004) Ill health is powerlessness: a phenomenological study about worthlessness, limitations and suffering. *Scandinavian Journal of Caring Sciences*, 18(2), 135–144.

Sturgess J (2003). A model describing play as a child-chosen activity: is this still valid in contemporary Australia? *Australian Occupational Therapy Journal*, 50(2), 104–108.

Sullivan M (2003) The new subjective medicine: taking the patient's point of view on healthcare and health. *Social Science and Medicine*, 56(7), 1595–1604.

Sunwolf Leets S (2004) Being left out: rejecting outsiders and communicating group boundaries in childhood and adolescent peer groups. *Journal of Applied Communication Research*, 32(3), 195–223.

Sussenberger B (2003) Socioeconomic factors and their influence on occupational performance. Chapter 8 pp. 97–110 In Crepeau E, Cohn E Schell B (Eds) *Willard and Spackman's Occupational Therapy*, 10th edition. Lippincott, Williams & Wilkins, Philadelphia, PA.

Taylor B Donnelly M (2006) Risks to home care workers: professional perspectives. *Health, Risk and Society*, 8(3), 239–256.

Taylor J (2000) Partnership in the community and hospital: a comparison. *Paediatric Nursing* 12(5), 28–30.

Taylor V Fuggle P Charman T (2001) Well sibling psychological adjustment to chronic physical disorder in a sibling: how important is maternal awareness of their illness attitudes and perceptions? *Journal of Child Psychology and Psychiatry*, 42(7), 953–962.

Thornton P (2003) *What Works and Looking Ahead: UK Polices and Practices Facilitating Employment of Disabled People*. Social Policy Research Unit, University of York, York

Todd S Jones S (2005) Looking at the future and seeing the past: the challenge of the middle years of parenting a child with intellectual disabilities. *Journal of Intellectual Disability Research*, 49(6), 389–404.

Tuckett AG (1998) Code of ethics: assistance with a lie choice? *Australian Journal of Holistic Nursing*, 5(2), 36–40.

Turner C (2006) *Fact Sheet 38. Adolescents with Tuberous Sclerosis Complex*. Tuberous Sclerosis Association, Birmingham.

Tweedale MG (2002) Grasping the nettle – what to do when patients withdraw their consent for treatment: (a clinical perspective on the case of Ms B). *Journal of Medical Ethics*, 28(4), 236–237.

Valkenier BJ Hayes VE McElheran PJ (2002) Mothers' perspectives of an in-home nursing respite service: coping and control. *Canadian Journal of Nursing Research*, 34(1), 87–109.

Walter T (1996) A new model of grief: bereavement and biography. *Mortality*, 1(1), 7–25.

Wang KK, Barnard A (2004) Technology dependent children and their families: a review. *Journal of Advanced Nursing*, 45(1), 36–46.

Watson D Abbott D Townsley R (2006) Listen to me too!Lessons from involving children with complex healthcare needs in resaerch about multi agency services. *Child:Care Health and Development*, 33(1), 90–95.

Whitehurst T (2006) Liberating silent voices – perspectives of children with profound and complex learning needs on inclusion. *British Journal of Learning Disabilities*, 35(1), 55–61.

Widdas D Sidey A Dryden S (2005) Delivering and funding care for children with complex needs. In Sidey A Widdas D (Eds) *Textbook of Community Children's Nursing*, second edition, pp 249–260. Elsevier, London.

Wilmot S (2003) *Ethics, Power and Policy: the Future of Nursing in the NHS*. Palgrave, Basingstoke.

Wilson S Morse J Pernod J (1998) Abslute involvement:the experiences of mothers of ventilator dependent children. *Health and Social Care in the Community*, 6(4), 224–233.

Wolfson L (2004) Family well-being and disabled children: a psychosocial model of disability – related child behaviour problems. *British Journal of Health Psychology*, 9(1), 1–13.

Wood JD Milo E (2001) Father's grief when a disabled child dies. *Death Studies*, 25(8), 635–661.

Worden JW (1991) *Grief Counselling and Grief Therapy*. Springer, New York.

Yantzi NM Rosenberg MW McKeever P (2006) Getting out of the house: the challenges mothers face when their children have long term care needs. *Health and Social Care in the Community*, 15(1), 45–55.

Zijlstra HP Vlaskamp C (2005) The impact of medical conditions on the support of children with profound intellectual and multiple disabilities. *Journal of Applied Research in Intellectual Disabilities*, 18(2), 151–161.

Index

abuse, children 136, 137, 138, 140
abuse, vulnerable people 93–94, 137, 138, 140
access
  to education 22–26, 94–95, 99, 107, 139, 178
  to facilities 19–21, 27, 90, 139
  to information 14, 80, 92, 117, 139, 153, 157, 158, 179
  to services 17, 92–93, 97, 139, 162, 175
accessing support 66–67, 117, 120, 158
adolescence 83–99, 178–179
advocacy 17, 36, 98, 133–136, 138, 140, 175, 179
advocate 98, 133–136, 179
assessment of need 2, 8, 49, 159–161, 161–162, 164, 166, 169, 173
attitudes 17, 27, 55, 56, 64, 66, 67, 87, 91, 92, 99, 110, 137, 167, 178
autonomy 61, 67, 87, 88, 122–125, 145, 147–148, 151, 153, 154, 155, 156, 179–180
  of child/young person 61, 87, 88, 122, 123, 125, 136, 148, 180
  of healthcare 125–127, 147–148, 151, 153, 154, 155, 156, 179–180

beneficence 145–146, 147
bereavement 100, 110
boundaries 60–63, 81, 135, 137

Carers and Disabled Children's Act 169
childcare, availability for children with complex health needs 42, 43
childcare practices 55, 57, 58, 69, 74, 75, 137, 176
child protection 80, 136–138, 140, 153, 178
Children Act 31, 49, 121, 122, 129, 136, 138

Children's rights 10, 11, 14, 18, 20, 22, 23, 26–7, 28, 31, 51, 58, 71, 121–122, 137, 165, 174, 175
Child's best interests 7–8, 55, 58, 121, 124, 129, 135, 141, 150
choices 12, 14, 17, 20, 22, 25, 27, 28, 38, 53, 77, 84, 88, 121, 122, 126, 127, 128, 132, 133, 134, 136, 139, 146, 150, 151, 156, 160, 168, 171, 173, 174, 175, 178, 179
chronic sorrow 102, 107
collaborative working 162–166
Common Assessment Framework 162, 165, 173
communication 11, 14–18, 20, 24, 25, 26, 27, 28, 33, 66, 84, 85, 89, 94, 98, 99, 101, 112, 115, 116, 117, 128, 130, 131, 133, 134, 137, 138, 140, 148, 162, 164, 166, 174, 175
competence
  consent 129, 130
  decision making 127–129, 130
complex health needs, definition 1–3, 174
concept of death: child/young person 112–115
confidentiality 26–27, 79–80, 82, 151, 153–154, 164
consent 80, 123, 124, 125, 127, 128, 129–131, 132, 138, 153
consistency in assessment 161–162, 173
consistency of support 12, 16, 59, 66,
co-ordination of services 8, 97, 98, 99, 162, 165, 166, 167, 173
cost, having a child with complex needs 7, 37, 42, 45, 46, 119

death 100, 108, 110, 112–115, 116, 117, 118, 119
  child's concept of 112–115

decision making 3, 7–8, 9, 12, 13, 14, 22, 27, 31,
    36, 37, 56, 57, 59, 67, 78, 85–86, 87–88, 97,
    107, 121, 122, 123, 125, 126, 127–129, 130,
    131, 132, 133, 134, 135, 140, 141, 142, 145,
    146, 147, 148, 149, 150, 153, 155, 156, 158,
    160, 162, 166, 174, 176, 179, 180
decision making, children and young people
    12, 13, 14, 27, 85–86, 87–88, 97, 121,
    122, 123, 125, 126, 127–129, 130, 131,
    132, 133, 134, 135, 140, 158, 160, 174,
    179, 180
demands on parents who have a child with
    complex needs 7, 38, 40, 41, 43, 44, 71,
    177
dependence on technology 3
developing relationship with
    child, parents 33, 35, 38, 39, 74, 177
    child, staff 12, 16, 52, 176
    families, staff 52, 53, 54–56, 57, 58, 59, 60, 61,
        62, 63, 64, 67, 69, 80, 168, 176, 177
diagnosis 2–3, 64, 80, 107, 111, 117, 118
dignity 10, 56, 78
Direct Payments 169–170
Disability Discrimination Act 23, 93, 138, 139,
    140
disability rights 23, 138–139, 140
duties of healthcare staff 58, 79, 89, 135,
    151–154, 155
duty of care 58, 77, 89, 154, 155

education 5, 22–25, 28, 34, 94–95, 99, 102, 103,
    105, 107, 138, 139, 140, 161, 165, 166, 175,
    178
employment
    parents 7, 26, 32, 42–43, 106, 119
    young people 94, 95–96, 97, 99, 103, 105,
        139, 178
empowerment 53, 62, 131–133, 134
equality 18, 22, 23, 24, 25, 53, 96, 138–140, 148,
    149
ethics 26, 55, 89, 141–156
European Convention on Human Rights 122,
    153
expectations
    child 103
    parents 31, 33, 34, 51, 52, 56, 57, 67, 68, 78,
        105, 106, 108, 159, 168, 176
    support 52, 56, 57, 67, 78, 159, 168
expert parents 35–37, 58, 63–66, 176
extended family 30, 49–50, 109–110

facilities for children with complex needs 21,
    42, 45, 91, 94, 103, 111, 175
family
    definition 29–30
    effects of a child having complex needs 7,
        42, 44–50, 176–177
    functions 29–30
fidelity 151, 154
Further Education 94–95, 99, 103, 178

grandparents 49–50, 81, 109–110
grief 100–120
    children 100–104
    extended family 109–110
    parents 104–109
    siblings 109–110, 112, 115
    staff 119–120
    theories 110–112

health and safety 77–78, 82, 178
health, definitions 11–12, 143
health needs and education 23, 24, 25, 94
holidays 12, 24, 42, 45–46, 109, 172
holistic 91, 130, 143, 149, 161, 162
home care
    challenges 7–9, 157–173
    economic issues 6–7, 167, 169–170
    evidence base: 4–9, 167, 170
    reasons for: 4–6
home, effects of needing care staff 41, 44, 45,
    53, 55, 56, 70, 71, 72, 73, 74, 75, 76, 81, 82,
    106, 159, 161, 162, 174, 176–177
Human Rights Act 122

impact of having a child who has complex
    needs 6–8, 21, 22, 24, 26, 29, 37–44, 44–48,
    49–50, 174, 176
inclusion 11, 23, 25, 139, 175
independence 19, 27, 28, 83, 87, 98, 99, 102,
    113, 130, 136, 139, 178, 179
independence, adolescence 83–86, 87, 98, 99,
    113, 136, 178, 179
independent funding options 169–170, 179
information
    availability 92, 93, 94, 127, 128, 133, 139, 157,
        158
    giving 66, 113, 117, 118, 126, 127, 128, 129,
        139, 148, 151, 152, 154, 155, 157, 158, 159,
        161, 173, 179–180
    sharing 64, 126, 153, 164, 165

intensive care units 4–5
interdisciplinary 164
intrusion 26–27, 44–45, 56, 62, 66, 69, 70, 71–76,
   81, 106, 117, 159, 160, 162
involving children and young people in
   decision making 12, 13, 28, 85–86, 88, 97,
   121, 122, 123, 125, 126, 127–129, 130, 131,
   132, 133, 134, 135, 140, 160, 167, 174, 175
involving families in decision making 31, 86,
   88, 97, 160, 174, 175

joined-up 161–162, 165, 166
judgemental 54, 55, 56, 58, 155, 180
justice 135, 145, 148–151

Key Worker 98, 99, 166–167, 173, 179

Lead Professional 98, 99, 179
legal aspects of care 78, 89, 121, 129, 130,
   142–143, 176
leisure activities 18, 20, 21, 27, 28, 90, 99, 103,
   175, 178
listening
   to children 12, 13, 28, 84–85, 99, 126, 128,
      132, 134, 137, 175, 179, 180
   to parents 65, 126, 180
living with loss 115–117
loss 33, 67, 100–120
   children and young people 100–104
   extended family 109–110
   parents 67, 104–109
   siblings 109–110, 112, 115
   staff 119–120
   theories 110–112

mainstream education 23–24, 25, 85, 90, 95,
   154
maternalism 132, 134
medical needs 24, 58–59, 63, 83, 87, 96, 163,
   165, 174, 176
morals 142, 143, 147
mother definition 31, 32
multiagency 164, 166
multidisciplinary 164
mutual respect 56–58, 76–77, 176

National Institute for Health and Clinical
   Excellence 149
national planning 148, 149, 179
need to be needed 62

needs assessment 2, 8, 161–162, 164, 166, 169,
   173
negotiation 52–54, 66, 69, 76–77, 81, 98, 145,
   146, 173, 177
neonatal intensive care 33, 34, 75, 126
neonatal period 146
NICE 149
non-judgemental 54, 55, 56, 58, 155
non-maleficence 145, 146, 147
nuclear family 30

opinions of child/young person 12, 13, 28,
   123, 124
organising support 8–9, 39, 157–173, 177, 178

paediatric intensive care 5, 6
parent, definition 29–31
parental responsibility 30–31, 57–58, 67, 69, 80,
   85–86, 123, 127, 160, 169
parenting 30–31, 58
parenting a child who has complex needs
   32–44, 176, 177
partnership 65–66
peers 10, 11, 12, 14, 15, 17, 19, 21, 22, 23, 24, 25,
   27, 28, 29, 62, 84, 87, 88, 89–90, 91, 99, 101,
   102, 103, 105, 118, 123, 130, 137, 171, 175,
   178
peer relationships in adolescence 11, 12, 17, 84,
   87, 88, 89–90, 91, 99, 178
play 18–20, 21, 22, 27, 28, 103, 104, 106, 114,
   115, 175
play facilities 19–20
potential, achieving 10, 12, 22, 167, 175
power 6, 13, 53, 62, 123, 131–133
   healthcare staff 6, 131–133, 134
   service users 6, 13, 53, 131–133, 134
preferences 10, 12, 13, 15, 16, 17, 27, 53, 61, 64,
   72, 77, 78, 139, 149, 159, 160, 168, 175
preparation for employment 94, 95–96
priorities 10, 12, 13, 16, 18, 20, 28, 31, 38, 39,
   55, 56, 58, 60, 64, 67, 68, 69, 87, 121, 124,
   130, 143, 159, 160, 162, 167, 168, 174, 175,
   176
privacy
   child or young person 26, 27, 28, 79, 80, 92,
      103, 136, 151, 152–153, 154
   family 33, 44, 71, 72, 73, 74, 79, 80, 81, 82,
      105, 144, 152–153, 154, 177, 178
   staff 76, 82
promoting health 142–145, 147

quality of life 3, 8, 9, 11, 12, 13, 28, 29, 34, 38,
    68, 85, 87, 88, 123–124, 127, 144, 147,
    159–160, 164, 173, 174, 179

redefining priorities 31, 38, 39, 106
redefining values 31, 39, 100, 106, 111
relationship between parents 31, 40, 43–44,
    79
relationship between staff and parents 52, 53,
    54–56, 57, 58, 59, 60, 61, 62, 63, 64, 67, 69,
    72, 80, 168, 176, 177
resource allocation 3, 6, 16, 25, 141, 144, 148,
    149, 151, 156, 159, 160, 172, 179, 180
respect 26, 27, 30, 54, 55, 56–57, 57–58, 59, 60,
    65, 66, 67, 69, 71, 76, 77, 79, 80, 91, 103,
    150, 151, 153, 158, 159, 160, 161, 163, 174,
    176, 180
responses
    to birth of disabled child 34–35, 104–105
    to loss, child or young person 100–104,
        110–112, 112–115
    to loss, extended family 109–110, 110–112
    to loss, parents 104–109, 110–112,
        115–117
    to loss, siblings 110–112, 115–117
responsibility and autonomy 154–155, 180
responsibility, parents 30–31, 52, 55, 57–58, 67,
    69, 80, 85–86, 119, 123, 127, 160, 169
rewards of having a child with complex needs
    31, 34, 37–38, 41, 51, 177
rights
    child 10, 11, 14, 18, 20, 22, 23, 26–27, 28, 31,
        42, 71, 121–122, 137, 158, 165, 174, 175,
        178
    parents 31, 50, 58, 66, 78, 82, 123, 127, 129,
        130, 140, 158, 165, 169, 176, 178
    staff 56, 77, 78, 82, 178
    young person 10, 11, 14, 18, 20, 22, 23, 26–7,
        28, 84, 86, 121–122, 137, 158, 165, 174, 175,
        178
risk 64, 77, 78, 82, 86–89, 99, 137, 145, 147, 148,
    153, 155, 160, 164, 178, 179
risk taking 64, 86–89, 99, 147, 179

self-awareness 62
self concept 90–91
self-determination 122, 126, 132, 134, 153
self esteem 27, 31–32, 36, 48, 90–91, 96
self image 90–91

sexual
    abuse 136
    expression 91–94, 138
    needs 91–94, 98, 99, 138, 178
sexuality 91–94, 138
short break services 161, 170–172
siblings 33, 45, 47–49, 75–76, 81, 137, 143–144,
    145
significant harm 58, 137
social life/opportunities, parents 32, 35,
    40–41, 73
social opportunities, children and young
    people 21–22, 84, 89, 92, 102, 103, 171
socialisation, adolescents 89–90
society, responses to children with complex
    needs 10, 17, 20, 21, 43, 47, 50, 51, 66, 67,
    90–91, 92, 99, 103, 108, 109, 110, 137, 176,
    177, 178
Special Educational Needs and Disability Act
    139, 140
staff
    recruitment 9, 59, 168, 170
    retention 59
    roles 53, 60, 61, 64, 65, 66, 69, 79, 117, 133,
        134, 135, 159, 168, 169, 177
    safety 76–79, 82, 178
state benefits 42, 66, 119, 157
stigma 38, 66, 108, 134
support
    definitions and types 157–159, 172
    emotional 158–159, 172
    enabling parents to access 66–67, 160–161
    groups 66, 157, 158–159
    information 66, 157, 159, 161, 172
    organisation of 157–173, 178–179
    practicalities 159, 167, 172
supporting families in loss 115–119
supporting young people 83–99, 178–179

technical needs 11, 25, 28, 35, 36, 63, 159, 174,
    176
technology dependent 3
theories of grief/ loss 110–112
time challenges for parents 32, 38, 39, 41, 161,
    162, 163, 167
transition
    to adult services 96–99, 179
    to parenthood 31, 32
transport to school/ college 25, 94, 95

trust 16, 58–59, 61, 64, 72, 80, 98, 118, 126, 151, 154
truth telling 118, 151–152, 155, 156, 157, 179

understanding of death, child/young person 112–115
United Nations Convention on the Rights of the Child 10, 14, 18, 22, 26, 42, 121, 122, 136

values
    definition 55
    individuals 10, 12, 14, 17, 18, 28, 30, 31, 38, 39, 54, 55, 56, 58, 60, 63, 64, 69, 71, 78, 83,
    87, 92, 100, 121, 124, 130, 133, 134, 135, 137, 146, 147, 150, 167, 175, 176, 180
    society 10, 14, 17, 19, 35, 36, 39, 43, 90–91
veracity 151–152
violence towards staff: 78–79
visitor in the workplace 70–71, 81, 162
vulnerable people 58, 93–94, 134, 140, 178

working in the family home 52, 53, 54, 56, 57, 63, 70–82, 153, 159, 169
working with parents 52–69, 117–119, 176, 177–178

young carers 49

Printed and bound by CPI Group (UK) Ltd, Croydon, CR0 4YY

09/06/2025

14685990-0001